UNLOCKING THE
KETO
CODE

ALSO BY STEVEN R. GUNDRY, MD

Dr. Gundry's Diet Evolution

The Plant Paradox

The Plant Paradox Cookbook

The Plant Paradox Quick and Easy

The Longevity Paradox

The Plant Paradox Family Cookbook

The Energy Paradox

UNLOCKING
THE
KETO
CODE

The Revolutionary New Science of
Keto That Offers More Benefits
Without Deprivation

Steven R. Gundry, MD

HARPER WAVE

An Imprint of HarperCollins*Publishers*

UNLOCKING THE KETO CODE. Copyright © 2022 by Steven R. Gundry. All rights reserved. Printed in Canada. No part of this book may be used or reproduced in any manner whatsoever without written permission except in the case of brief quotations embodied in critical articles and reviews. For information, address HarperCollins Publishers, 195 Broadway, New York, NY 10007.

HarperCollins books may be purchased for educational, business, or sales promotional use. For information, please email the Special Markets Department at SPsales @harpercollins.com.

FIRST EDITION

Designed by Nancy Singer

Library of Congress Cataloging-in-Publication Data has been applied for.

ISBN 978-0-06-311838-6

22 23 24 25 26 LSC 10 9 8 7 6 5 4 3 2

To searchers and researchers, whose purpose is to always question conventional wisdom, including our own.

CONTENTS

UNLOCKING THE
KETO
CODE

CHAPTER 1

HOW WE GOT
KETOSIS WRONG

Spoiler alert! How ketones work is not how you think they work. With so many things, what's old is new again. While the ketogenic, or "keto," diet, has been around since the 1930s, there's been a resurgence of interest in this high-fat, ultra-low-carb way of eating in the past few years. Talk to your friends, surf the internet, or scan the nutrition articles in your favorite magazine, and you'll see many variations on the keto theme. There's dirty keto, clean keto, calorie-restricted keto, high-protein keto, the Paleo/keto hybrid, keto cycling, protein-sparing keto, and even a lazy man's version of this popular dietary regimen. Its proponents will tell you that this eating plan is life-changing—do keto "right," whatever that means, and you'll soon find yourself not only shedding unwanted weight quickly but improving your cholesterol, blood pressure, energy levels, and sleep quality in the process. Who wouldn't want all that?

While each type of ketogenic diet has its own unique quirks, the premise of them all is basically the same—and, as it so happens, deceptively simple, and wrong. Keto experts will tell you that when you drastically reduce your carbohydrate intake and instead consume 80 percent of your daily calories from fat, your body shifts into a unique metabolic state called ketosis. In ketosis, the liver transforms fats into special molecules called ketones (sometimes referred to as ketone bodies), a so-called miraculous fuel source that can be used to power the body and brain instead of glucose that comes from carbs. The basic idea is that a ketogenic diet will make you an incredibly efficient fat burner, allowing you to rapidly lose weight and enjoy a host of other health benefits. Sounds great, right?

This very elementary explanation of ketosis (don't worry, I'll go into more detail in the following chapters) has been the presiding theory of why ketogenic diets, though challenging to maintain, are so beneficial to well-being. In my first book, *The Plant Paradox*, I even put forth my own keto-based intensive care program to help people boost mitochondrial function and improve their overall health in the process. It's the diet I've been prescribing to my own patients for the past twenty-two years.

There's only one problem: ketones are not the miraculous cellular fuel that so many of us thought they were. We now understand they actually aren't a good fuel source at all. In fact, the entire theory of how ketones improve health is just plain wrong. That's not to say ketones aren't important. As I'll explain in the following chapters, these little molecules play a vital role in helping to ease the burden of your mitochondria, your cells' energy factories, in ways that can help prevent as well as reverse not only weight gain but also diseases of aging. Even more important? Once you learn what ketones really do, you'll realize you don't have to force yourself to eat a heavy, high-fat, and, frankly, boring diet to harness their power.

A TALE OF TWO PATIENTS

Janet, a forty-three-year-old mother of two, came to my Palm Springs clinic for help after her family physician diagnosed her as prediabetic. Her resting blood sugar, or glucose level, was higher than the normal range—but not yet high enough to be considered full-blown type 2 diabetes. Her doctor wanted to start her on a statin drug for high cholesterol and revamp her diet in order to right the ship, so to speak. That brought her to my door.

After running my standard battery of tests, I agreed with her doctor that she had metabolic syndrome, a cluster of health issues that can increase one's risk of cardiovascular disease and diabetes, as well as insulin resistance, a condition where your body actually *resists* the insulin your pancreas produces so your cells can't get the vital glucose they need to thrive. As you'll soon learn, Janet, like nearly all Americans, was metabolically inflexible. Sounds bad, right? It is. The tests also showed signs of excess inflammation. But I didn't see a reason to start her on the statin. I thought we could manage her issues with diet and I suggested she try my Plant Paradox Keto Intensive Care Program.

Three months later, Janet came back into the office for new lab tests. We found that she had lost 15 pounds and her blood work showed she was no longer prediabetic. Shockingly, at least to her primary care doctor (but certainly not to me), her cholesterol had also improved to the point where, according to her regular doc, a statin was no longer necessary. Needless to say, Janet was delighted. She felt more energized and was sleeping better—and, like many of my patients, she was motivated to keep going. We eased up on the high amount of good fats I had recommended she eat to promote ketosis and scheduled a follow-up appointment.

When Janet returned six months later, she was down another 20 pounds and her lab work looked spectacular. Her blood tests showed no signs of inflammation and her HbA1c, a measure of how well controlled your blood sugar is, was down to 4.9 (anything under a 5, in my opinion, is worthy of a literal gold star). In short, Janet's case presented as a perfect keto success story.

Except for one thing: Janet was not happy. She, like me, was pleased with her test results. But despite the fact that she was eating like a horse, concerned friends were commenting that she looked a little *too* thin. Even as she added different foods back into her diet, her weight continued to fall. She told me she was ready to stop losing pounds and stabilize.

Let me tell you that Janet is not the only person who has experienced this phenomenon. Many of my patients have gotten to a similar point with my eating plan where they actually had trouble keeping their weight stable. Given common wisdom regarding ketogenic diets, I told them, as I told Janet, that they had simply metamorphized into extremely efficient fat burners. I know you might be thinking, "What are they complaining about? I wish I had that kind of problem!" Follow some food rules, take a few supplements, and get to a point where you want to gain a few pounds? It sounds like a dream come true.

Now contrast Janet's story with that of another patient of mine. Miranda came to see me around the same time as Janet—and the similarities didn't end there. She was also a busy mom in her forties. But unlike Janet, she was obese. Her previous doctor had suggested she go on a ketogenic diet a few years prior. She had been trying to follow the traditional keto diet to the letter, yet she was not only unable to shed any of her excess weight, she had actually added more than 15 pounds over the course of a year. The more fat she ate, she told me, the more weight she gained.

Miranda came to see me because her primary care physician, the one who had recommended she go keto in the first place, didn't believe she was following the diet correctly. This is quite common: often, when ketogenic diets don't deliver the promised results, the assumption is that the dieter isn't eating enough fats to trigger ketosis (and is, perhaps, sneaking in too many carbohydrates and/or protein foods). This presumption, for the most part, is not meant to question the integrity or will of the dieter. We know our patients are working hard. But traditional ketogenic diets—and this is one of their biggest downsides—are extremely challenging to maintain, especially over time.

I gently explained to Miranda that despite her best efforts, it was clear that whatever she had been eating (or not eating) hadn't helped her body make ketones. She was shocked, even apoplectic, to hear this. I softened the blow by saying she was like many of the people who come to see me after struggling to eat the keto way. They *thought* they were on a ketogenic diet—but they simply weren't getting enough of the right fats and other foods you will learn about in this book they needed to reach ketosis.

Miranda then showed me the food diary she kept. By most keto standards, she was doing things perfectly. About 80 percent of her calories were coming from fat. But when we looked at her blood work, we saw that she, unlike Janet, had an HbA1c result in the prediabetic range. (It should be noted that the National Institutes of Health report that 1 in 3 Americans are prediabetic and, if the condition is not corrected, will go on to develop type 2 diabetes later in life.) Her fasting insulin levels were high, indicating that she was insulin resistant—that is, her body was no longer responding to insulin the way it is supposed to, letting that insulin build up to high levels in her blood. And as we already know, she just saw the numbers on the scale continuing to rise.

Miranda's story is one that is also well-known to me. Many people come to my clinic after failing to lose weight on some form of ketogenic diet. They are frustrated and confused, and wonder why so many people can find success eating this way, but they can't.

I should add that there is a third category of patients that comes to my clinics. These folks are intrigued by the idea of a ketogenic diet for weight loss, but they simply can't stomach the idea of eating all that fat. They also tend to question how healthy such a diet, with such harsh restrictions on plant-based foods, can be over the long term.

Over time, seeing these different people getting such different results raised some important questions. How could folks like Janet see such health gains accompanying weight loss while other people, like Miranda, have blood work that indicates declining metabolic health?

It's a conundrum. You may well be wondering what the difference is between the Janets and the Mirandas of the world. With both on a keto regimen, how can one woman follow the rules (and even eventually relax those rules) and lose so much weight, while the other follows the same guidelines and gains weight? At the time, I would have told you it had to do with the types of fats the two women were eating—Janet's focus on more plant-based fats and proteins, as opposed to animal-based ones, was helping her body become a more efficient fat-burning machine. But those differences don't tell the whole story. In fact, as I studied the matter further, I soon learned something absolutely incredible: the conventional keto wisdom about metabolic efficiency and fat burning was flat-out *wrong*. The production of ketones actually results in your body becoming more fuel inefficient. Those molecules should help your body *waste* calories, and they do so through your cells' mitochondria. What's more? You don't need to consume a diet of 80 percent fat to reach that level of inefficiency.

LESSONS LEARNED FROM IDENTICAL TWINS

Any time a physician sees two patients respond differently to the same intervention, it can be easy to attribute the outcome to some sort of innate difference in their physiology that cannot be easily observed—perhaps it's their genes! Yet in a recent study comparing sets of identical twins in which one sibling was overweight and the other was not, researchers discovered something fascinating: though the twins shared an identical genome, they did not metabolize calories the same way. In fact, the heavier twins' mitochondria, or cellular energy factories, were less active than those of the thinner twins. The researchers even referred to their mitochondria as "lazy"! (It's important to note that this does not in any way mean the heavier twins themselves were lazy. Rather, their mitochondria simply weren't getting the signals required to nudge them into picking up the pace. We'll talk more about those signals later.)

If you struggle with your weight, as many people do—45 percent of Americans are obese—the blame does not lie with your willpower, your "fat" genes, or your family history. Instead, it has everything to do with your mitochondria and how hard they're working. Their job is to burn the calories you eat, and when they lay down on the job, those calories stick around and get stored as fat. This begs the question: How can you jump-start those sluggish mitochondria so they'll start picking up the slack?

Common wisdom suggests you have two choices. You've likely heard, ad nauseam, that you need to eat less and exercise more. The other option is to go "keto" to rev yourself into a fat-burning machine. Yet for some people, like Miranda, the latter doesn't work out so well. Why is that?

We all have that one skinny friend who seems to eat anything and everything they want without gaining an ounce. Meanwhile, others, like me and perhaps you, so much as look at a croissant, even after completing an energetic Spin class, and still see the scale numbers creep up. It would seem like those skinny twins, as well as those skinny friends, have a way of just making any calories they consume magically disappear. Here's the shocker—and the reason for this book: they *do*. As you'll soon learn, the skinny folks of the world have mitochondria that literally waste a huge number of the calories they eat. That's right: *waste*.

Remarkably, Janet got to the point where the pounds melted off her body by eating in a way that kicked her mitochondria into gear. The best part? It didn't require a diet composed of 80 percent fat. She didn't have to force down a pound of bacon with a shredded cheddar cheese chaser to stay in ketosis. She simply had to give her mitochondria the signals required to get them to open up their membranes and let those calories just pass on through—a process called *mitochondrial uncoupling*. She wasn't becoming a more efficient fat burner, as I had told her so earnestly back in the day. She was, in fact, becoming the exact opposite: a fuel waster.

IT'S NOT WHAT YOU THINK

This book reveals a new and incredible paradox regarding ketones and their role in weight loss, health, and longevity. As I mentioned, it turns out that they aren't some special source of magic cellular fuel. Rather, they are vital signaling molecules that tell your mitochondria to get up, get moving, and start wasting calories.

Our mitochondria produce fuel for our bodies by taking glucose, amino acids, and fatty acids from the foods we eat (which your gastrointestinal system has so kindly broken down from carbohydrates, proteins, and fats, respectively) and converting them into a special molecule called adenosine triphosphate (ATP), an energy "currency" our cells can actually spend.

But the latest research shows that mitochondria are involved with much, much more than just energy production. They play an integral role not just in survival, but longevity. Yet to truly understand what mitochondria do—and why ketones are produced, when they are produced, and their ultimate purpose—you need to let go of everything you thought you knew about keto.

If you're familiar with The Plant Paradox or any of my other books, you likely know I'm famous (or perhaps infamous) for challenging people's long-held beliefs about "healthy" foods. Disruption is in my nature. Even in my previous career as a heart surgeon, I pushed back on the way things had always been done, discovering new ways to protect my patients during open-heart surgery that are today considered best practices in care. Now, just like Mark Antony in Shakespeare's famous play, I come not to praise keto, but to bury it—at least the conventional notions of the keto diet (or even most so-called healthy diets, for that matter).

The best part? When you understand the role of mitochondria and how they affect your metabolism, you no longer have to worry about fat percentages, macronutrient proportions, calories, or any other metrics. This new understanding provides a healthy path forward for folks like Janet, Miranda, and even all the people who have wanted to try a keto approach but couldn't get past the fat requirements. And that's because, as you will learn in the following chapters, the role of ketones in weight loss and health is not what you think—and harnessing their benefits doesn't require you to consume massive amounts of saturated fats. Intrigued? Let's get started.

CHAPTER 2

KETONES ARE NOT A SUPER FUEL

True story: While researching and writing my last book, *The Energy Paradox*—a look at how we can enhance mitochondrial energy production and, in the process, boost our energy levels—I came across some startling information about ketones. These molecules, long lauded as an incredible cellular energy source, weren't actually meeting the body's metabolic needs. That raised a vital question: If ketones weren't providing an alternative fuel source for the body and brain, just what were they doing—and to what end?

I found myself falling down a rabbit hole of data. After reviewing the latest research over and over again, I discovered the true function of ketones—and it had been there in plain sight all along. Despite the fact that I've spent more than twenty years practicing restorative medicine, I, like many of my colleagues, couldn't see the forest for the trees. Once I opened my eyes, I saw clearly that ketones don't work as an incredible fuel, but instead unlock the vital molecular process known as mitochondrial uncoupling, and that this phenomenon underlies everything we didn't know about how to support health, well-being, and longevity.

I am well aware that my findings may be considered heretical by advocates of ketogenic diets. I expect some pushback from the individuals who have found success on a keto program, whether by shedding excess weight or correcting various health problems. That includes many of my own patients, who happily dropped a few pants sizes, not to mention saw their overall health dramatically improve, after adopting the ketogenic versions of my programs.

My goal in this book is not to suggest that we forget about ketones altogether, but rather to challenge the traditional notions we've held about their role in the body and share what I've learned about how they influence mitochondrial health. Once I understood what we'd gotten wrong about keto, it became clear to me that my patients were harnessing the power of ketones without having to eat a traditional high-fat ketogenic diet, just as Janet did. In fact, the data suggests eating a conventional keto diet may even be harmful to long-term health in some cases, as we saw with Miranda.

As we move forward, I'm going to ask you to suspend your current beliefs about what it means to be "keto." I will challenge you to open your mind and think bigger and bolder. You're going to finally understand why all those diets you've tried, keto and otherwise, didn't deliver on their promises. But before we look at how to do things right, we first need to review what we got *wrong*. To start, let's take a closer look at ketones.

WHAT ARE KETONES, ANYWAY?

These water-soluble (meaning they dissolve in water) short-chain carbon compounds were first identified in Germany in the 1880s in the urine of diabetic patients.[1] At the time, they were considered little more than a symptom of metabolic disease. But just a few decades later, doctors in France and the United States who happened to be researching epilepsy in children stumbled across a rather amazing discovery. When epileptic children were given a diet composed of 80 percent fat, 10 percent protein, and 10 percent carbohydrate, the frequency and severity of the seizures was significantly reduced. For some children, this protocol stopped the seizures altogether. The only other dietary intervention that even came close to that level of effectiveness was a water fast—meaning the children consumed nothing but water for 18 to 24 hours at time to keep the seizures at bay. As you can imagine, forcing growing children to abstain from food simply wasn't a feasible or humane long-term option.

Physicians were stymied as to the mechanism at work, but the results were clear: the diet was an effective treatment for at least 50 percent of youngsters who could not find relief from their seizures by any other method. But why? Why would a high-fat diet (or, for that matter, a lack of any food at all) reduce seizures?

Fast-forward to 1921, when an endocrinologist at Northwestern University named Rollin Turner Woodyatt made a surprising discovery while researching diabetes. Woodyatt found that the body doesn't just produce ketones as a result of metabolic disease. Instead, he discovered, the liver produces ketones when an animal is either starved or consuming a diet rich in fats but restrictive in protein and carbohydrates. The liver does this by picking up free fatty acids (FFAs)—lipids that come directly from the fats we produce and store in our fat cells—and converting them into ketones. Woodyatt's research identified three distinct types of ketones: acetone, beta-hydroxybutyrate (BHB), and acetoacetate (AcAc).

Less than a year later, Dr. Russell Wilder, a pioneering researcher in diabetes and nutrition at the Mayo Clinic, used Woodyatt's discovery to develop a high-fat, low-carb diet that he called a "keto-genic diet"—and used it to treat children with epilepsy. In these young patients, the diet didn't just help to control seizures; it also improved sleep quality and seemed to increase the children's energy. The ketogenic diet became the standard line of treatment for child-hood epilepsy for years, until antiseizure medications like phenobar-bital and Dilantin came along.

It's worth noting that the ketogenic diet reemerged as a favored treatment for epilepsy in the 1960s, with proponents recommending a diet with high amounts of medium-chain triglyceride, or MCT, oil, a special type of saturated fat that is metabolized differently than other types of fats. This form of the diet still helped to control sei-zures, but without excessive fat consumption, allowing the patients to enjoy more protein and carbohydrates. If you're asking yourself, "How could that work?"—hold that thought. We'll come back to MCTs and how they influence the formation of ketones, and the role they play in my Ketogenic Intensive Care Program in *The Plant Paradox*.

WHAT WE THOUGHT KETONES DID

When you put all the research together, it becomes clear that ke-tones are generated in three different ways: during feast (high-fat diets), during famine (starvation), and in the presence of diabetes (metabolic disorder). What is the tie that binds all three?

The short answer: carbohydrates. The body converts carbohy-drates into glucose, which our mitochondria then use to make ATP, the energy that powers our cells. Insulin helps to usher glucose into our cells, but when diabetics lack sufficient insulin, either because their bodies no longer make it (type 1 diabetes) or become resis-tant to this hormone (type 2 diabetes), their bodies have difficulty making ATP. On the other side of the spectrum, if you're starving or eating a carbohydrate-restricted diet, your body doesn't have access to the glucose it needs to make ATP. Given the importance of glucose for keeping our bodies gassed up and ready to work, that raises an important question: Just what might be working as an alternative fuel for making ATP when glucose is unavailable?

When food is unavailable to us, our cells first turn to glycogen, the form of glucose stored in the liver and muscles, to keep us going. But what happens when that is used up? In the 1960s, seminal work by Dr. Richard Veech, a biochemist and medical doctor by training, finally answered that question. Veech discovered something interesting while exploring the nuances of human metabolism. Researchers already knew the liver produces ketones during fasting or while following a high-fat, low-carb diet. Veech, in partnership with his mentor, Dr. George Cahill, a diabetes expert based at Harvard University, discovered that one type of ketone body, beta-hydroxybutyrate (BHB), could not only stand in for the absent glucose to help generate ATP but also kicked off a number of downstream effects that had nothing to do with energy production. They hypothesized that BHB, as well as other forms of ketones, might be an alternative fuel source. (It's those downstream effects, as I later learned, that really give ketones their power. But let's get back to the history lesson.)

This finding led Veech and Cahill to hypothesize that ketones are produced by the liver as an alternative fuel source when carbohydrate-rich food sources are scarce. After all, our bodies need energy to run. Heck, our brains alone use 20 percent of our body's total energy production. Veech and Cahill theorized that in order to survive in times of insufficient glucose availability (famine), the body would burn existing fat, releasing FFAs to be converted into ketones. The body would then use ketones to produce the energy it required. They even argued that ketones were a form of "super fuel"—a source of cellular nourishment that could make cells (brain cells, in particular) work even better than plain old glucose could.

After all, our forebears had to find food where they could, even during the cold, dark winter months. Having the ability to use ketones instead of glucose to meet their energy needs prevented them from dying when the hunting was poor or the fields lay fallow. This fail-safe system meant our bodies, unlike those of many animals, were well built for any circumstance. We could gorge ourselves when food was relatively easy to find or grow, but we could also make do during droughts and periods of famine. Having an alternative fuel source ensured our bodies could function, perhaps even perform at a higher level, to help us stay alive until we were able to hunt down the next gazelle or forage for the next tuber.

Today, it is still widely believed that ketones are a brilliant insurance policy that helps us survive tough times. Some ketone advocates will even go as far as to say ketones are miraculous—an incredibly efficient form of "super fuel" for our brains and bodies. In the past, I was one of those keen proponents, suggesting to patients like Janet that their weight loss was the result of their having become a super-efficient fat burner. And yet, I, like so many of my peers, fundamentally misunderstood how ketones work. Ketones may perform miracles, but not in the way we all believed they did.

HOW WE THOUGHT KETOGENIC DIETS WORKED

When the first ketogenic diet was prescribed more than a century ago, there was no real understanding of how it helped with seizures—or patients with other types of neurological disorders. It worked and that was all that mattered.

Dr. Veech was the first scientist to credit BHB with enabling ancient humans to survive when food was unavailable. It was a theory that made some sense: by switching to this alternative metabolism during starvation, early man could live significantly longer than he could on glucose, provided by carbohydrates and protein, alone. And when Veech's research proved that humans continued to make ATP even when abstaining from food for weeks, it seemed to tie everything up in a nice little bow. (In fact, we now know that humans can survive for quite a long while without food—for instance, in 1971, Angus Barbieri, an extremely obese British man, successfully completed a 382-day water-only fast under medical supervision—yet the side effects of extensive fasting are quite dangerous, and include increased strain on the heart, muscle deterioration, and malnutrition. This is not a healthy path to weight loss or longevity.)[2]

The ketogenic diet is predicated on the idea that when there's no glucose to be had, the body needs to turn to stored fat for fuel. After fasting for about 12 hours (remember this number, please!) or restricting carbs to 20 grams or less a day, assuming you aren't insulin resistant, the FFAs released when fat breaks down can serve as an alternative fuel source for most cells in your body. However, those FFAs can't fuel your energy hog of a brain. You may know that the brain is protected by a special network of tissues called the blood-brain barrier. It's there to keep the bad stuff away from this precious organ—only certain substances, which include water, sugar, and oxygen, can pass through easily. Other molecules, particularly larger molecules, get turned away. That's why FFAs can't help your brain cells. They are simply too large and not water-soluble enough to quickly cross the blood-brain barrier and get to where they are most needed.

Let's be clear: when you're starving, most of your cells switch over to using FFAs as fuel instead of glucose. But your brain can't partake of these molecules. So how can it get the fuel it needs to make energy? We now understand that a few of the FFAs released from your fat cells arrive at the liver, where they are converted into ketone bodies (another term for ketones)—which are smaller and water-soluble, meaning they, unlike FFAs, can easily cross the blood-brain barrier to get into the brain. There the ketones can be used as "emergency" fuel for your brain cells, helping the mitochondria in your neurons produce the ATP they need to stay in top working order. (Fascinatingly, while ketones are made in the liver, the liver can't actually use them as fuel. They dump them out into the bloodstream.)

Okay, so far, so good. The liver makes ketones. Ketones can go to the brain to be used as fuel when glucose is lacking. And if Veech is correct, every cell in the body (except those in the liver) can receive and then leverage this "most excellent" energy source. If that's the case, we should strive to be in ketosis 24/7—and essentially always be starving—right? Our bodies will burn fat and make ketones, and every organ and system will be happy. Well, excuse the pun, but not so fast!

Dr. Oliver Owen, another protégé of George Cahill's at Harvard who studied diabetes and human metabolism, challenged that notion in the late 1960s when his research uncovered that ketones only provide up to 70 percent of the brain's total energy requirements. When humans fast for a prolonged period, not only do our muscles start to deteriorate—our brains can and do suffer as well. That means that even when the body is fully operating in a state of ketosis, the foundation of the ketogenic diet, ketones simply cannot replace all the glucose the brain demands to function at its best.[3]

Owen and Cahill found yet another wrinkle in Veech's "super fuel" theory. While ketones were the preferred fuel source for muscles during a three-day fast, their study participants switched to burning FFAs after twenty-four days of fasting. Ultimately, after a host of additional studies, Owen broke the news to the scientific community: ketones are not a sufficient energy source to keep the body and brain running at optimal levels. In fact, in 2004 he demonstrated that only about 30 percent of the body's energy-production needs can be met by ketones during full ketosis.[4]

Think about what you just read. Even when your body is generating tons of ketones, the brain isn't satisfied with this so-called miracle fuel. It wants—no, it *needs*—glucose. Your muscles aren't fully satisfied by ketones, either. They will use them for a while, sure, but after a time, they'll switch to FFAs. And then, even if you can max out your ketone production, less than a third of your body's total energy needs will be met.

This raises the question: How is it, exactly, that experts are still suggesting that ketones are a superior form of metabolic fuel, one that we should strive to make and use instead of glucose?

A KETOGENIC DIET FOR WEIGHT LOSS

You may have noticed that neither Veech, Cahill, nor Owen had much to say about weight loss, per se. How did doctors and scientists shift from focusing on ketones as a source of energy to promoting a ketogenic diet for weight loss? I'll tell you.

As doctors used the ketogenic diet to treat epilepsy, they noticed something interesting. People on high-fat diets tended to lose a lot of weight—and lose it fast. This result flew in the face of the prevailing nutritional science at the time, which suggested that the logical result of eating a high-fat diet could only be weight gain.

Then, in 1972, Dr. Robert C. Atkins, a cardiologist, published *Dr. Atkins' Diet Revolution*. The book was inspired by the runaway bestseller *The Drinking Man's Diet*, a treatise written by a photographer named Robert Cameron that described the benefits of a low-carb, high-animal-protein diet (with a lot of alcohol thrown in for good measure). This fad diet essentially banned the consumption of carbohydrates. While Cameron's book was largely considered bunk by physicians and nutritionists at the time, Atkins thought there was something to the idea of limiting carbohydrates.

Atkins noticed an alarming trend with his cardiac patients: they were increasingly suffering from obesity. He recognized the link between this extra weight and cardiovascular issues—and blamed excessive carbohydrate intake for America's expanding waistlines. He soon developed what he called a "controlled carb approach" to weight loss, championing the consumption of protein and fats, including saturated fats, instead of the cereals and grains that covered the typical plate. While Dr. Atkins did not refer to his weight loss program—which limited carbohydrate intake to 20 grams a day and eschewed most grains, vegetables, and fruits—as a ketogenic diet, he did argue that eating this way allowed the body to use fat instead of glucose for energy.

In the decades since *Dr. Atkins' Diet Revolution* was published, the eating program was modified to include more vegetables, fruit, and other complex carbs as a person got closer to their weight loss goal. However, both in the Atkins diet and the numerous imitators that followed it, the reality was that the weight loss (and, more often than not, maintenance of that weight loss) lasted only as long as the carbohydrate restriction was in place. Once someone began to eat a more balanced diet, the weight usually returned, often along with an extra 5 to 10 pounds. Indeed, multiple studies in humans bear testimony to the fact that while a low-carb, high-fat "keto" and/ or a high-protein diet usually promotes more rapid weight loss and correction of insulin resistance than low-fat diets, the effect wears off quickly. In fact, when Danish researchers from the University of Copenhagen directly compared the long-term health effects of these various diets, they found few differences in the results observed after the course of a year.[5]

Yet, today, as we all know, the ketogenic diet has made yet another resurgence. Its premise, like that of any other carb-restricted diet, is that it forces the body to make ketones and then utilize them for fuel, prompting a quick and "magical" form of weight loss. How does it do this?

Dr. Atkins believed that ketones in the urine represented lost energy that helped to promote the shedding of all those pounds. Other purveyors of high-fat diets have suggested that this might work because ketones somehow "waste" calories, leading to the loss. (As it turns out, these folks are right, just not for the reasons they think!) Still others have promoted the idea that ketones might suppress the appetite or, as demonstrated in research by David Raubenheimer and Stephen Simpson, leading experts in nutritional ecology from the University of Sydney, that eating this way makes you feel full faster, so you ultimately eat less.[6] And then, of course, there remains the popular theory that ketones somehow help the body become more efficient at burning fat, making short work of both the fats you eat as well as existing fat in the body. This is what I used to believe—after all, I did tell Janet she had become a remarkably efficient fat burner.

Regardless of the fact that the medical community didn't really understand how ketosis and weight loss were related, most popular ketogenic diet books didn't hold back from making bold claims. In fact, here's a sampling of quotes taken directly from some of the biggest keto "experts" out there (names have been omitted to protect the innocent!):

- "You are burning fat for fuel and weight loss will be effortless."
- "Ketones are merely a by-product of burning fat for fuel."
- "Ketones are actually the body's preferred source of fuel."

- "Ketones are the most efficient fuel."
- "Ketones are a clean fuel and glucose is a dirty fuel."
- "Ketones are actually the perfect fuel source for muscles, heart, liver, and brain. These organs do not handle carbohydrates very well."
- "You can become keto adapted in a few days."
- "Ketones are the fourth macronutrient, the fourth way of making ATP."
- "Up to three-quarters of the world's population is carbohydrate intolerant."

No wonder so many people want to try a ketogenic diet. (Or think they might like to try it, if it didn't involve eating all that fat!) Reading these claims, you may be inspired to cut out carbs tomorrow yourself. There's only one problem: ketones are not a great fuel. In fact, everything most experts thought they knew about ketosis and weight loss is utterly wrong.

THE DOWNSIDES OF A TRADITIONAL KETO DIET

After highlighting all those incredible keto weight loss claims, I'd be remiss if I didn't mention that there are quite a few drawbacks to a ketogenic diet. To start, not all carbohydrates are created equal. Both Swiss chard and a brownie are considered carbohydrate-containing foods. One of those foods is chock-full of phytonutrients (plant-based nutrients like polyphenols) and fiber. The other is decidedly not. A long-term eating plan that severely limits how much carbohydrate you can eat makes it almost impossible to get the nutrients your body needs to live optimally.

And that is because—as I've long advised in my books and with my patients—your overall well-being is largely dependent on the health of your microbiome, the population of bacteria and microbes that reside in the human gut. Without a diverse and abundant supply of fiber, polyphenols, and nutrients in the form of vegetables and other plant foods, your microbiome can't get the raw materials it needs to help you thrive.

When all carbs are considered equal, significant nutritional differences between different varieties of fruits, vegetables, and grains—including how each of these foods impacts your metabolism—also get ignored. For example, simple carbs like sugar and refined grains are digested much more quickly than complex carbs like fibrous veggies, properly prepared beans, and nuts. Carbs, as a category, cast a wide net, and include all manner of junk foods right alongside members of the plant kingdom.

There's another downside to strict carb restriction that needs to be addressed. While some keto experts will tell you three-quarters of us are "carbohydrate intolerant," that statement is pure nonsense. All animals have a need for carbohydrates. Animal brains even have an innate sensor to help make sure we get enough of carbohydrates, so our bodies will have the glucose they need to make ATP and survive.[7]

In addition to the carb confusion that results from going keto, these diets pose other significant challenges:

- **High fat content.** As someone well-known for saying that the only purpose of food is to get more olive oil into your mouth, I'm certainly pro-fat, but a keto program that indiscriminately allows all fats is not a healthy approach. In chapter 6, we'll delve into the significant differences among dietary fats.
- **High cholesterol content.** If you adhere to the cholesterol theory of coronary artery disease—meaning high cholesterol is to

blame for heart disease—the long-chain fats that are consumed in a traditional ketogenic diet almost always raise LDL cholesterol, which may send your local healthcare provider reaching for their prescription pad. While I don't happen to agree with this theory, my program shouldn't cause your LDL numbers to shoot up.

- **Animal fat and protein.** For most vegans and vegetarians, the traditional keto diet is a nonstarter because plant protein sources tend to contain carbohydrates. That makes it a big challenge to comply with the traditional keto diet's demand for 10 percent content with regards to both carbohydrate and protein energy sources. Other people prefer a plant-based diet for health and/or ethical and environmental reasons.

- **Boredom.** The need to significantly restrict the intake of even healthy carbohydrate foods can make for monotonous meals. This is undoubtedly a big reason 60 percent of people don't manage to stick with a keto diet for even a short period of time.[8]

- **Questionable athletic performance.** Some studies suggest that being in ketosis does not impair performance, but the data is mixed. In *The Art and Science of Low Carbohydrate Performance*, low-carb researchers Jeff S. Volek and Stephen D. Phinney conducted a number of experiments with athletes, the results of which suggested that a high-fat diet wasn't detrimental to performance. However, even they concede that athletic performance tanks initially and that it may take weeks to get "keto adapted." In other, more recent ketogenic diet experiments, researchers discovered elite race walkers could retain their peak performance on a high-fat diet, but doing so required more oxygen (in other words, they had to breathe harder and faster) to produce the same amount of ATP than when they were consuming a more carbohydrate-rich diet. In these elite athletes, at least, carbohydrate is able to produce a greater ATP yield per unit of O_2 consumption than fat. This presents a bit of a problem for the traditional notion of keto: if ketones really were the super fuel that so many suggest they are, you would think you'd see athletic performance skyrocket, not fall, or at least stay relatively unchanged.

- **Increased inflammation and heart disease.** If you can achieve a near constant state of ketosis—and that's a big "if," by the way—you may actually be putting your health at higher risk. A joint study conducted by Columbia University and the NIH demonstrated that eating a keto diet was linked not only to higher cholesterol but increased inflammation across the body. What's more, it appeared to make subjects who followed the diet *more* insulin resistant, despite all those promises about it helping to regulate metabolism![9] Just this week, one of my more zealous keto practitioners was shocked to see these very issues present in his own blood work.

Let's say you can overcome these obstacles and make keto work for you. Most keto experts promise that the production of ketones will make you an efficient, fat-burning machine! But consider that claim for a moment. Merriam-Webster defines "efficient" as "capable of producing desired results with little to no waste." If ketones are truly making your body more efficient at burning fat, you should be making more energy with less fuel. A hybrid vehicle like a Toyota Prius is definitely a more efficient fuel-burning machine than, say, a sports car like a Ferrari. You can travel about 50 miles on a single gallon of gas in a Prius. That Ferrari, no matter how good-looking it is, will give you somewhere around 10 miles per gallon. So, if I wanted to use up a lot of gas—to literally waste it—I'd pick the Ferrari.

(Okay, there might be other reasons I might want to tool around in the Ferrari, but let's stay with this efficiency analogy.)

Carbs and protein contain about 4 calories per gram. Fat, on the other hand, contains about 9 calories. That's more than twice the calories! So if you're eating mostly fat, with double the calories by weight of what you used to eat, you shouldn't be losing any weight. Those excess calories should be going straight to fat. After all, as an efficient fat burner (or one who burns body fat to produce more energy), you should have extra calories in spades and, as a result, pack on the pounds more easily.

In other words, if ketones were making me an efficient fat burner, they would make me like a Prius, a very efficient fuel burner. And that would make me use less fat, not more. On the other hand, if I wanted to waste fuel (fat), I'd jump in the Ferrari, a very efficient fuel waster indeed. This is the essence of the keto conundrum: when the keto diet is working, it appears that it is doing exactly the opposite of what its proponents say—it appears to be making people and their mitochondria profoundly fuel inefficient!

I need to mention one other thing. In a new meta-analysis of high-fat ketogenic and/or modified Atkins-style diets, researchers could not only find *no* benefit with regard to weight loss when it came to this style of eating, but also did not see any form of type 2 diabetes reversal. In fact, these researchers found that this type of diet led to increased inflammation and risk factors for heart disease. It's yet another example that keto, at least as it's currently understood, is not the healthy option so many keto evangelists tell you it is.[10]

So, fat-based diets are not helping you become a more efficient fat burner, despite what I and many other keto proponents once might have thought. That's why Miranda and so many other patients I see experience the opposite of all the keto promises. The efficient-fat-burning explanations of ketogenic diets just don't hold up.

TIME TO LOOK AGAIN

Roughly 80 percent of the people who arrive at my clinics looking to slim down claim to either be following a ketogenic diet—or, like my patient Miranda, to have valiantly tried such a program without success. Despite ketogenic diets being all the rage, the sad truth is that very few people actually achieve the desired results. On the surface, it would seem that they simply aren't following the program properly.

But I knew there had to be something else going on that was preventing people from achieving success on a keto diet. In my early days as a research fellow at the NIH, my mentor, Dr. Andrew G. Morrow, would often say, "There is nothing new to learn. But there's lots to *relearn*." Dr. Morrow defined research as "to look again; to literally *re*-search."

Thanks to his influence, I actually look for reasons I might be wrong about something. As I pored over mitochondria-related research with the goal of explaining how these energy-producing organelles work, I realized that instead of serving as a fuel, ketones act as *signaling molecules*, sending critical messages to our mitochondria, the energy-production factories in our cells. This may seem like a subtle difference to you—a footnote in a scientific paper—but there is a profound difference between these two functions. The prevailing theory suggests that ketones serve as the high-grade gasoline that makes our bodies run smoothly and efficiently. As shown earlier, however, they are not anywhere close to a super fuel. But in their role as a messenger, they tell mitochondria to "uncouple" and literally waste fuel to protect themselves from too much work. This groundbreaking new understanding of ketones can unlock your potential not only for weight loss—but for vibrant health.

Once you know how the foods you choose to eat can help you harness the power of your mitochondria, you'll find you can and will improve your weight and health, all while slowing the aging process. You'll never look at "keto" the same way again. Even better? This new science supports a dietary program that is much more permissive, enjoyable, and sustainable than traditional keto diets—no need for all that fat!—with even better results.

You are, no doubt, excited to learn more. But as in all my other books, before we get to the program itself, a little basic knowledge on our subject is required. It's time to revisit how your mitochondria work and why their well-being is so critical to yours. Let's get going.

CHAPTER 3

HARNESSING OUR CELLS' PETITE POWERHOUSES

You may remember mitochondria from studying the anatomy of the human cell in eighth-grade biology class; they're the tiny, rod-shaped organelles that live inside almost every cell of your body. Mitochondria have a very important job: they produce energy. While your middle school textbook diagram may have shown a token two or three mitochondria floating in the cell's cytoplasm (for simplicity's sake), in reality, most human cells are packed with them. In fact, the majority of your body's cells contain anywhere from 1,000 to 2,500 mitochondria.[1] I can't give you a more specific estimate because the number can change at any given time based on your health status and activity level. But what I *can* tell you is that you'll find larger numbers of mitochondria in the cells that make up your muscles, brain, heart, and liver, as these are the tissues and organs that have the biggest jobs in the body and therefore require the most fuel.

Mitochondria produce energy by converting glucose, amino acids, and fatty acids from the foods you consume into ATP. I know I've used this analogy in my previous books, but I always picture mitochondria as little clones of Mighty Mouse, the superhero from the classic 1950s cartoon. I used to love to watch Mighty Mouse use his super strength and invincibility powers to "save the day" when I was a kid. Your mitochondria, like that mouse, may be minuscule, but they are mighty. And they save the day by producing the energy your body needs to function.

Chances are—unless you're a student cramming for a biology exam—you don't think much about mitochondria these days. After all, their work is both silent and invisible. Yet believe me when I tell you the effort required to produce all that ATP is herculean. The human body has staggering energy demands. An average-size person in good health is estimated to make somewhere around 140 pounds of ATP each day.[2] You read that right—*pounds*. If you consider that as a fairly conservative estimate, you probably eat somewhere in the neighborhood of 3.5 pounds of food a day, that's a tremendous return on investment. (If you're thinking, "Wait—I only weigh 140 pounds! How is that possible? Where does all that ATP go?" the answer is simple: your body's cells spent it. And that's just at rest. When you're active, your cells' energy demands are much, much higher.)

Is it any wonder mitochondria are referred to as the powerhouse of the cell?

AN EVOLUTION IN ENERGY PRODUCTION

Mitochondria have a fascinating history. The prevailing theory of their origin is that they evolved from engulfed bacteria. If you rewind back to two billion years ago, the world was full of different types of bacteria—but some other fledgling types of cells were also in the mix. As the story goes, one of those cells, likely a precursor to the eukaryotic cells that make up most of life on earth, engulfed one of those bacteria. They started to work together, forming a symbiotic relationship from which both organisms benefited. The bacterium helped the cell to respire, or use oxygen to make energy. The cell, in return, gave the bacterium a home, helping to keep it safe from the elements. Over millions of years, the bacteria within those cells evolved into mitochondria.

Despite the fact that mitochondria exist inside our cells, they've never fully given up their bacterial roots—they are actually quite similar to the gut bacteria that inhabit your microbiome. In fact, just like your "gut buddies," as I like to call them, mitochondria have their own DNA. They can divide at the same time as their host cells divide, but they can also divide to make more mitochondria at any time they please via a process called mitogenesis. Their ability to replicate themselves without the rest of the cell having to divide is critical for you, your health, and your fate, as you will soon discover.

Today, your microbiome and mitochondria are still tethered by their shared bacterial past. They stay in touch via signaling molecules called postbiotics, which, generally, are produced by the microbes in your gut—although many of them are also present in some of the foods we eat. Your gut microbes vigilantly monitor everything that takes place in your body. They're in a great position to do the job, as they regularly receive information about the state of affairs from both your immune system and your nervous system. They then pass along messages to the mitochondria via postbiotic signaling molecules, communicating how much energy is needed. These messages range from "Hey, we have a big workout today, let's crank up production!" to "Uh-oh! I think we ate something rotten. Let's shut things down until we figure out what's going on." How much energy is being produced by your mitochondria is largely influenced by the information they receive from your microbiome. That's another reason traditional keto diets, which restrict plant-based fiber, can lead to side effects like fatigue and brain fog. That fiber is essential to a thriving microbiome. A thriving microbiome, in turn, produces postbiotics. We'll discuss this in more detail soon, but first, let's take a closer look at how our energy factories work.

HOW MITOCHONDRIA MAKE ENERGY

The technical name for the conversion of food and oxygen into energy is *cellular respiration*. It's a process that occurs over and over again in every single mitochondrion in the body—and, if you recall, your body houses trillions upon trillions of mitochondria. You can think of cellular respiration as a bit like an internal assembly line. It takes multiple steps to convert glucose to ATP.

As any *Star Trek* fan can and will tell you, human beings are carbon-based life-forms. We also consume carbon. All the food we eat, whether it's made up of sugars, amino acids, or fats, eventually breaks down into a bunch of carbon molecules. Those carbon molecules make their way inside the cells where they are scooped up by the mitochondria to kick off the energy-production process. This is the start of the Krebs cycle (sometimes called the citric acid cycle), the series of reactions that turns those carbon molecules into ATP. (As an aside, Hans Krebs, the scientist who first described this cycle, and won a Nobel Prize for his discoveries, was the mentor of Drs. Veech and Cahill. But I digress.)

Once the carbon molecules pass into the mitochondria, they begin a fascinating dance with protons and electrons, some of which come from water. You may recall that these are charged (think electrified) particles. The protons carry a positive (+) charge and the electrons carry a negative (–) one. Those protons and electrons are then ushered across the inner mitochondrial membrane into the innermost part of the organelle. There they go through a series of chemical reactions known as the electron transport chain. It's complex stuff—but, simply explained, that chain helps to ramp up the charges of those particles. As the charge increases, the excited electrons and protons become proverbial hot potatoes, becoming hotter and hotter as they jump from one level of charge to the next.

Things are so "hot" in this situation that you can think of this process a bit like a bunch of twentysomethings heading out for an evening at the latest, greatest night spot. Imagine a single mitochondrion as the hottest new club in town. Let's call it the Mito Club. This hip spot has one main entrance that lets in patrons and a one-way revolving door at the rear through which they can exit. (There are also some emergency exits. The Mito Club does want to stay in code, after all, but we'll talk more about those later. At this point, there's only one way in and one way out for the Mito Club's patrons.)

The Mito Club is steamy, crowded, and packed to the gills with hundreds of protons, electrons, and other molecules like oxygen and hydrogen. Because the Mito Club can get so full—anyone who is anyone is trying to get in—a doorman oversees the entrance. It's his job to only admit so many. But even with the doorman working hard, patrons can barely get to the bar without bumping into at least a dozen other people. And just like at a real club, there are plenty of protons and electrons who are there with the hope of connecting (coupling) with an oxygen molecule.

Some manage to couple with that desirable oxygen. They link arms and head to that back revolving door—and make a lot of ATP upon exiting. It's a bit like how water creates power when it turns a mill wheel. When the positively charged protons, now coupled with oxygen, pass through the mitochondria's membrane, they together make some of that much-needed energy currency. (Furthermore, in the process of exiting, the protons leave behind carbon dioxide, or CO_2. In this scenario, you can think of CO_2 as the beer bottles and other trash the proton patrons are tossing before heading out the door with their dates.)

It's a typical jam-packed Saturday night when all of a sudden, a lot of the electrons decide they've had enough and are going to leave. They've been lured away by the promise of a good time elsewhere, perhaps with an oxygen molecule or two. That leaves a bunch of protons, who had hoped to connect with some oxygen themselves, milling about and realizing that the odds of connecting with that lovely oxygen is quickly diminishing. The frustrated protons see the Exit sign in the distance and now make a beeline for the door.

At the exit, some of those protons may meet up with some wayward oxygen molecules and finally manage to couple up. Then, as these new couples push through the revolving door, they produce the high-energy molecule ATP. But most of the other protons won't be so lucky. They are going to exit the club alone and unfulfilled. They won't be making any ATP tonight.

I should mention that this process isn't quite as simple as I just made it sound. Remember, it's hot in the Mito Club, with protons, electrons, and other molecules all slammed up against each other. As you can imagine, those conditions can lead to some pushing and shoving. When the doorman realizes trouble is brewing, he'll call in his bouncers to deal with the drama and let the protons couple up with oxygen in peace. In actual mitochondria, this multistep process of trying to combine oxygen with protons to make ATP can lead to more than just the production of some CO_2. The coupling of these different particles and molecules can also lead to the production of some potentially nasty pollutants called reactive oxygen species (ROSs). Think of ROSs a bit like the exhaust from your car's engine. In the Mito Club analogy, I think of them as the patrons who have overindulged and start throwing punches. The bouncers will eventually deal with them but that doesn't mean that they don't cause a ruckus!

You see, sometimes, when electrons end up coupling with oxygen instead of the protons, ROSs, which include the free radicals that we health experts talk about so much, are produced. These ROSs create oxidative stress, which damages the mitochondria and, as a consequence, the cell. You've probably heard of ROSs and oxidative stress before. Both have been implicated in aging and chronic disease.

Now, some ROSs are okay. The Mito Club wouldn't be the place to be if there wasn't a little excitement. That whiff of danger can be quite intoxicating, after all! In small amounts, they act as signaling molecules, sending messages to help keep your cells healthy. It's only when ROSs are produced in excess that they become a problem. Your mitochondria can be damaged when too many electrons and oxygen molecules couple up. Even worse, if the Mito Club's bouncers don't find a way to keep the ROSs in check, they can induce apoptosis—literally the cell's explosive and immediate death. Too many fights, too much drama, and the club would have to be shut down.

The Mito Club's two main bouncers are melatonin (yep, that sleep hormone and antioxidant you've heard so much about) and glutathione, a lesser-known but critical antioxidant. They help keep those ROSs in their sweet spot: just enough of them milling about to perform their signaling duties, but not so many as to harm the cell. As you can imagine, the Mito Club likes to have plenty of those bouncers to make sure things don't get out of hand. (In the following chapters, you'll learn that you actually have more control of ROS production than you might think.)

BUT WHAT ABOUT KETONES?

The club analogy offers a brief summation of the Krebs cycle and the electron transport chain (ETC). When molecules from the food you eat and the oxygen you breathe arrive at your cells, the mitochondria couple these ingredients together to generate ATP. Mitochondria can process sugars, amino acids (from proteins), and free fatty acids (from dietary fats) into energy. Oxygen plays a pivotal role in the making of this energy currency. But it also has the potential to damage and even destroy mitochondria—the oxidative stress of energy production takes a toll. That's why your mitochondria shift to a slow burn at night. They use those slower production hours to take it easy and do any necessary repair work. (That's also why so many people who suffer from insomnia also tend to be overweight—getting enough sleep is vital to mitochondrial health.)

Consider it this way: if the club opens each night at six and closes at two a.m., there is plenty of time to clean up the place. There's a whole 16 hours to deal with spilled drinks, discarded trash, and whatever else the ROSs have left behind. Now, imagine that the club expands its hours from ten in the *morning* to four a.m.—the poor cleaning crew gets a measly six hours to tidy up! Pressed for time, the crew will be forced to cut some corners. The floor will still be a little sticky, garbage will start to pile up. Pretty soon, the Mito Club is going to become a dingy place where no one wants to go. When you shorten your sleep cycle, your mitochondria are in the same boat. They won't have time to clean up, repair any damage, and get back into top working order!

Do you know what stimulates this necessary repair downtime? The appearance of free fatty acids and ketone bodies. That's right— with no new food to process, the mitochondria make a shift. They start using the fat stored in your fat cells, built up from all the left-over sugar, protein, and fat you didn't use during the day, as a signal that it's time to clean up the Mito Club. When food consumption stops, these stored fats are released into the blood as free fatty acids. You can think of them as your slow-burn energy.

Under certain conditions, your mitochondria, particularly those residing in your brain cells, can *also* use ketones as a fuel source. Generally speaking, this occurs when sugar supplies stay low for a significant block of time. This may be because you (1) have been following a ketogenic diet, restricting the amount of carbs and proteins you've consumed; (2) have fasted for a period of about 12 hours; (3) burned up all your stored sugar (glycogen) through some seriously intense exercise; or (4), worst-case scenario, are literally starving. Just to be clear, ketones play a key supportive role in mitochondrial health. But as we've discussed, that role has been misunderstood.

In some ways, our energy production system mimics that of a hybrid car. When the car is running on gasoline (glucose), the battery is being recharged (fat storage), and this stored energy can be drawn upon once you've used up the gas or turned off the engine altogether. At night, when you aren't eating for a period of 8 hours or more, mitochondria draw on that battery power, in the form of free fatty acids or ketones, to make the ATP you need.

CROWD CONTROL

The Mito Club is only designed to hold a certain number of patrons at any given time. There's the fire code to consider, after all. But sometimes, a larger crowd than anticipated comes into the joint. Like when you eat a large meal. The club, representing one of your mighty mitochondria, tries desperately to keep up with all the people coming through its doors, working hard to allow protons and oxygen molecules to couple up so it can convert glucose into energy. Unfortunately, especially with today's typical diets, the Mito Club just can't keep up with the crowd.

You can probably guess what happens next. When your mitochondria are forced to simultaneously juggle ATP production with storage, all while protecting themselves from those potentially damaging ROSs, energy production slows down while fat deposits go up.

Now, if the club only became overly crowded occasionally, it wouldn't be such a big deal. After all, even our hunter-gatherer ancestors sometimes found themselves in a period of plenty and would enjoy a big feast to celebrate. Your mitochondria can easily handle a bit of excess from time to time. But when that number of entrants continues all day long without a break, your mitochondria are going to suffer. There's got to be a better way. A plan B, if you will, for the Mito Club.

Upon first consideration, it may seem like the best approach is simply to limit how many patrons can enter the club. Maybe the doorman can just throw one of those classy velvet ropes in front of the door, letting the crowd form a line to wait outside. Restricting access may seem like the obvious answer, but it doesn't account for insulin, the hormone produced by your pancreas to help you metabolize carbohydrates. Insulin shunts sugars and proteins out of your bloodstream and into your cells. It essentially knocks on the cell wall and asks if the cell wants or needs any glucose or protein.

That velvet rope should give your mitochondria some much-needed time to catch up on the backlog—but only if you stop eating. If more and more digested food continues to enter your bloodstream, your pancreas will release more insulin, creating an army of insulin molecules to tell your cells to open up and let in the patrons who are there to couple. The Mito Club doorman, however, will not yield to all that knocking. The end result? You'll have less energy getting into the cells, energy production will significantly slow, and blood sugar stores will build up. Insulin levels will rise to try to correct the problem—but the line outside the club door will grow longer and rowdier.

Over time, this problem only worsens. If you have read a keto book or two, you may think, "Well, surely the FFAs from your fat cells, as well as ketones from your liver, can get into the cells without insulin's help." Fats and ketones don't require insulin to get into the cells, so they can restart energy production—and they're just sitting in all those storage spaces (your fat cells) waiting to be used. But here's the cruel gut punch, if you'll pardon my word choice: the presence of insulin tells your fat cells to hang on to their fat stores.

There is some evolutionary rhyme and reason for this blocking action: when your ancient forefathers were able to feast on that recently felled bison or newly discovered ripe berries, they needed their insulin levels to rise in order to help save those sugars and proteins by ushering them into fat cells. Thus, they needed any fat-liberating action to be put on pause during those times of plenty so the body could save those extra carbs and proteins for a rainy day. If you're trying to store fat, it would be crazy to simultaneously have someone else unloading the storage unit.

Think about it. Typically, if your insulin level is high, it means you've eaten recently. You've got the calories you need to make your energy! If there's any extra glucose hanging around, it should be stored, not used. So after all that, simply stated, insulin not only helps you to process carbohydrates, it also blocks your body's ability to liberate stored fat.

When you have a normally functioning, flexible metabolism, your insulin levels fall as soon as you stop eating. With insulin now low, FFAs can flow out of your fat cells and into the waiting arms of the mitochondria that need fuel. Your liver will be prompted to make a few ketones to help tide over your brain until the next meal. Unfortunately, far too many of us are now metabolically inflexible. We eat too much, our insulin levels are always high, and, as a result, we have ample stores of fat but no way to release them for use.

This is why you'll find that when embarking on an ultra-low-carb or high-fat ketogenetic diet, your metabolism will initially sputter to a stop. Your energy levels tank, your brain feels foggy, and you just feel, well, awful. Whether you call it the "keto flu" or the "Atkins blues," this state is the result of high insulin levels blocking fat release and, consequently, the production of ketones. Even though most keto diets promise that your body will start making ketones as soon as you restrict carbohydrates, this is, quite frankly, impossible if you have developed insulin resistance—which is why my patient Miranda was never able to lose weight on keto. Like so many other people who have had a frustrating experience with this diet, her insulin levels were simply too high to allow her fat stores to be released.

That said, even if you are insulin resistant, it is possible to make the transition to liberating fats, allowing your body to use them as fuel. I'll teach you how to do that shortly. Here's a hint: the secret lies in the messages ketones send to your mitochondria.

IT'S TIME TO UNCOUPLE

While today, many use the term *uncoupling* to describe leaving a romantic relationship, mitochondria have their own way of divorcing the burning of fuel (metabolism) from the production of energy (ATP). Let's talk about *mitochondrial uncoupling*. Uncoupling is truly the key to unlocking the keto code—and it offers benefits far, far greater than just weight loss.

Let me explain how uncoupling works using the Mito Club analogy. As you know, this juke joint is *the* place to be, and the line to get inside has just gotten long and longer. Things are getting hot inside and, at a certain point, your protons are no longer interested in coupling up with some oxygen—they want to leave and either try a new place or call it a night. The Mito Club has just that one exit at the back. With the crowd in there, the door is easily bottlenecked. But then someone pushes open one of the emergency exits nearby. Bam! The patrons rush out the side door, so invigorated by their new freedom that they head down the block to try their luck at "coupling" somewhere else.

Now that some capacity has opened up, tension dissipates and patrons can enjoy themselves again. In fact, those protons and oxygen molecules now have room to start coupling up again. Furthermore, the doorman can now admit some of those folks who have been waiting outside. But within just a few minutes, the club is jam-packed again. What should the owner do? He's got unhappy customers—both those who are packed tight inside and those outside waiting to enter. He needs a new game plan.

With so many patrons milling about outside with nothing to do, it's clear the cell could use another club or two (mitochondria) to keep up with demand. In the cell, we call this process mitochondrial replication, or mitogenesis.

Under certain circumstances, your cell will literally make more mitochondria to handle the workload (as you may recall, they have their own DNA and can divide when they need to, regardless of what the rest of the cell may be doing). Most experts will tell you there are only two ways to make more mitochondria: fasting and exercise. But I'm here to tell you there are several other ways to invoke mitogenesis. With the right signals in place, instead of adding to your fat storage, you can subtract from it.

So the club owner decides to build more clubs. He's perfected a recipe for success with the Mito Club. But to create those new venues, he needs a bank loan. Where does he go to get that kind of cash? He can tap the fat stores to provide the resources to build the new clubs (mitochondria) and start producing all that feel-good energy again.

Okay, you might be thinking, "But why would the fat stores give out their currency? Didn't you just tell me that most people can't get the fat out of storage due to insulin resistance? Something isn't adding up." You'd be right in thinking so. It takes the involvement of unique proteins, nudged by ketones, to open up those side doors, promote mitogenesis, and tell the fat stores to open up.

UNCOUPLING FOR HEALTH

In 1978, physiologists David Nicholls, Vibeke Bernson, and Gillian Heaton, researchers at the Buck Institute for Research on Aging, discovered that mitochondria have built-in "emergency exits" for the different players participating in the electron transport chain. Those exits are controlled by uncoupling proteins.[3]

Today, we know there are five total uncoupling proteins, UCP1 to UCP5. They all reside within the inner mitochondrial membrane and allow protons to exit under certain circumstances. Like the Mito Club patrons sneaking out the side door, our mitochondria can allow uncoupled protons to leave the cells' energy-producing power plants—and waste calories in the process!

Ketones, as well as other molecules we will discuss in later chapters, send messages to the mitochondria to open up those emergency exits, or uncouple, so they make less ATP than they could potentially make. In the process, the mitochondria perform a caloric bypass, literally *wasting calories* instead of using them for fuel.

You may wonder why producing ketones—something that will lead to you wasting perfectly good fuel—could possibly be a good idea when your body thinks it's starving. No doubt, it is counterintuitive. But as we'll soon discuss, our mitochondria "uncouple to survive." As first described by Martin Brand, PhD, a prolific researcher who studies the mechanisms of energy transformation in the human body, mitochondrial uncoupling is all about protecting the mitochondria themselves.[4] Additionally, mitochondrial uncoupling produces heat through a process called thermogenesis. That heat plays a significant role in weight loss, vitality, and optimal health. (And, consequently, may explain why Drs. Veech and Cahill were so convinced that ketones were some sort of "miracle fuel.")

Are you ready to get started? In the following pages, I'm going to teach you how to leverage mitochondrial uncoupling to waste fuel and thrive while doing so. Unlocking your mitochondria will set them free—along with those extra pounds you've been trying to lose.

CHAPTER 4

THE POWER OF UNCOUPLING

You now understand that the process of mitochondrial uncoupling can help your cells waste fuel—and kick-start your metabolism in the process. In fact, research shows that in a normally functioning body, mitochondria waste about 30 percent of all incoming fuel. Thirty percent?! What reason could Mother Nature possibly have to waste so much perfectly good energy?

In biology, things tend not to happen without a very good reason, and in this case, Mother Nature knows exactly what she's doing. As I mentioned previously, one side effect of mitochondrial uncoupling is thermogenesis, or the generation of heat. Warm-blooded animals like ourselves use uncoupling to keep our body temperatures in the proper range. In many animals, that job is relegated to what is called brown fat, which gets its color from being packed to the gills with mitochondria. Brown fat has a special purpose: it produces heat. Studies now show it does so via uncoupling.[1]

Let's return to the Mito Club for a moment. Making ATP is hard work. As electrons are pushed around by the crowd, they can sometimes end up coupling with some unsavory characters, resulting in the creation of reactive oxygen species (ROSs) and free radicals. These rogue actors can build up over time and damage the mitochondria. Get enough of them together, and they could destroy the Mito Club outright, or at the very least make it into the kind of establishment no one wants to frequent.

The emergency exits for the Mito Club function a lot like the release valve on a pressure cooker. When you can uncouple and send some of those protons away, you can create more space, venting some of that pent-up pressure, so things don't get out of hand. After all is said and done, animal life—including your life—depends on healthy, well-functioning mitochondria. For that reason, any mitochondrial building code should require not only those emergency exits but also make sure to have plenty of bouncers on hand for those occasions when the atmosphere gets a little too charged.

Remember: The emergency exits are located within the mitochondria's inner membrane. The bouncers? Those are the antioxidants melatonin and glutathione. You may be thinking, "If these antioxidants are good for our mitochondria, I should get more antioxidants into my body!" You wouldn't be the first to think so. For years, we believed we could simply swallow a few antioxidants like vitamin C and vitamin E to help protect our mitochondria from oxidation. Easy enough, right? Take some supplements or pick up the latest "superfoods," and voilà, you've protected your cells from damage. Unfortunately, this just isn't the case.[2] (As an aside, in 2014, I had the pleasure of presenting a paper at the World Congress on Polyphenol Applications, held in Lisbon, Portugal. At the opening of the conference, the chairman of the organization, Dr. Marvin Edeas, addressed the thousands of researchers present at the meeting by saying, "Anyone who thinks that polyphenols work as antioxidants may leave the room right now. I don't have enough time to bring your knowledge into the twenty-first century!" Stay tuned—we will talk more about polyphenols and how they influence and protect your mitochondria in the coming pages.)

If you can't just swallow more bouncers, what can you do to protect this vital piece of cellular real estate? As it turns out, more than you might think. This is where the dots start to connect, demonstrating the key to health and wellness that has been hiding in plain sight all this time. This is where we see just how powerful mitochondrial uncoupling can be.

Unlocking the Power of the Fab Four

I like to refer to the quartet of ketones, butyrate, other short-chain fatty acids (SCFAs) and postbiotics, and polyphenols as the Fab Four. They all, in their own uncoupling fashion, help to keep your mitochondria in first-rate shape. Let me share one more really nerdy downstream effect of this group of molecules: they all act as histone deacetylase inhibitors (HDACis)! I know—that's a mouthful. But you don't need to remember the name or even the acronym. What you need to remember is that these are all cancer-fighting agents.

You see, cancers use histone deacetylases to help them grow and invade your organs and tissues. When you have molecules that can inhibit that action, like the Fab Four, you can hinder, or even altogether prevent, cancer cell growth. Beyond being cancer fighters, HDACis also play a role in helping to support your mitochondria, signaling that it's time to protect themselves, not to mention the cells they inhabit, when times get tough.

As a heart surgeon, I studied another HDACi known as valproic acid.[3] This incredible molecule actually protects the heart and brain during circulatory arrest. When we do certain types of open-heart surgery, we have to literally stop the heart and blood flow for up to an hour to do the necessary repairs. Valproic acid, yet another uncoupler, ensures that we can start things back up with ease.

Valproic acid is also used as an antiseizure drug. Coming full circle here, remember that the ketogenic diet got its start as a treatment for epileptic seizures in children. Behold the power of mitochondrial uncoupling! The Fab Four, as well as valproic acid, all uncouple to protect and defend your cells, organs, and body.

TOO MUCH OF A GOOD THING

Let me tell you a story about a prescription weight loss drug that was used by hundreds of thousands of Americans in the 1930s. During World War I, many munition plant employees in France and Germany displayed an interesting side effect of their jobs. Despite eating huge amounts of food, these workers couldn't seem to keep weight on. They were all painfully thin. They seemed to be running a temperature as well. What was going on?

Investigators soon learned that 2,4-dinitrophenol (DNP), a compound used to make explosives, was the culprit. (Please note the "phenol" in that compound, and file that thought for later.) Sensing an opportunity, Drs. Windsor C. Cutting and Maurice L. Tainter at Stanford University decided to test DNP as a potential treatment for obesity. Their work showed that consuming DNP—literally swallowing it—led to the same significant weight loss seen in the European munitions workers.[4] Consequently, it was soon marketed as a miracle weight loss drug and prescribed to more than one hundred thousand Americans alone—and thousands more worldwide.[5]

And DNP worked. Boy, did it work! People who took only a small dose could lose a pound a week. At an increased dosage, some patients reported weight loss in the range of 5 pounds a week. It was incredible. Researchers wanted to know how it worked its magic. Further studies showed that DNP somehow increased the basal metabolic rate, resulting in patients burning more calories from the food they ate, as well as burning the calories from their existing fat stores. The end result? A lot of weight lost very, very quickly.

Sounds like a wonder drug, right? You may even be wondering where you can get a prescription. Unfortunately, the DNP story turns sinister fairly quickly. The more DNP people took, the more weight they lost, certainly—but there were soon repeated reports of very high temperatures, thyroid issues, cataracts (this was long before cataract surgery was possible), and even deaths. The pounds may have been melting off, but people who took DNP were getting quite sick in the process. Then, in 1938, the Food and Drug Administration (FDA), in one of its very first acts, deemed the drug a threat to public health and banned its sale.

Drs. Cutting and Tainter had no way of knowing how DNP worked. It wasn't until Nobel Prize–winning biochemist Peter Mitchell discovered the mechanisms of ATP production in the late 1970s that researchers understood why DNP-fueled weight loss was so dangerous. As it turned out, DNP was the first oral powerful mitochondrial uncoupler to be discovered.

FINDING SOME BALANCE

Wait, I can almost hear you saying, "Given DNP's terrible side effects, should I even want my mitochondria to uncouple? Losing some weight sounds great, but I have no interest in those other health consequences. Maybe performing that kind of caloric bypass on my mitochondria is actually counterproductive. Shouldn't we want to make more energy, not less?"

In *The Energy Paradox*, I refer to the Goldilocks Rule when it comes to energy: you don't want too little or too much of a substance that stresses the body—you want the "just right" amount. You can probably guess where a high dose of DNP falls when judged by this rule. It's way too much. The Goldilocks Rule is how I define hormesis, the biological process by which a seemingly harmful substance can actually be beneficial in small doses. What if the things we typically think of as stressors—like limited fasting, heat, and cold—actually lead to mitochondrial uncoupling? That could explain the paradox of their effects—and why mitochondrial uncouplers can improve an organism's longevity.[6]

Let's think about the Goldilocks Rule in terms of the Mito Club. By opening the emergency exits, the club was able to defuse a potentially volatile situation that could have shut down the place for good. Clearly, uncoupling was beneficial. But—and this is a big "but"—unless you have a way to compensate for having fewer customers, you can end up with a long-term problem for your business.

That compensation comes from building more clubs (translation: making more mitochondria). If you don't make more mitochondria and fuel is just wasting away, you have no hope of maintaining the ATP production an organism needs to survive, let alone thrive. That was the problem with DNP; it uncoupled mitochondria but did not help people make more of them. Losing energy via caloric bypass without having a replacement to make more energy is a recipe for disaster. That's something many DNP users found out too late.

BUT WHAT ABOUT KETONES?

"All right," you might say, "you've convinced me that DNP is a terrible idea, but DNP shows what uncoupling can do for weight loss. I need to find ways to uncouple my mitochondria while somehow signaling my cells to make more of the little buggers. How do I make that happen?" If you said ketones, you'd be right on the money.

I've already explained that ketones aren't the miracle fuel that so many claim they are, and that they can uncouple mitochondria. But they also participate in another vital process: mitogenesis. That's right, ketones send signals to instruct your mitochondria not just to start wasting calories and slow down ATP production, but also to make more of themselves to take up the slack.

Let's go back to the basics. Your liver makes ketones from free fatty acids (FFAs) when you're starving—when your food intake does not provide enough glucose to make energy. Ketones don't completely replace that fuel. Rather, they signal your mitochondria to uncouple, thus making *less* energy, even when resources are scarce. Why in the world would any organism waste precious fuel in this manner when you don't know where your next meal is coming from?

It's yet another paradox—and elegant in its simplicity. In extremis, the only thing worth saving are your mitochondria. Your body can suffer a lot of losses on the cellular front, but if all the mitochondria die, the entire organism will eventually run out of energy. No energy, no life. So the longer you remain in ketosis, the harder your mitochondria work to save themselves. Forget about catering to those energy-hungry muscles.[7] Not your mitochondria's problem! Instead, your mitochondria will use all the available energy to produce more of themselves, adding workers to the assembly line to keep up with ATP production while simultaneously protecting themselves from damage. And they do so by wasting fuel.

The Goldilocks Rule, however, applies here as well. Sadly, as a good friend of mine, an osteopathic physician, learned while experimenting with an extreme 24/7/365-day version of the ketogenic diet, your mitochondria can protect themselves *too much*—and, in the process, fail to produce proteins required for your muscles. By staying in ketosis for such an extended state, his muscles became profoundly wasted—a medical condition known as sarcopenia. That's something to avoid.

But what if you could experience the benefits of a ketogenic diet without the drawbacks? What if you could find a way to uncouple those mitochondria, wasting all those calories, without having to force down a diet made up of 80 percent fat? Without having to be in ketosis 24/7—which is an extremely challenging thing to do? Given that ketosis is such an effective way to lose weight, wouldn't you jump at the chance?

You absolutely can.

Consider this: What do the following items have in common?

Ketones	Fermented foods
A 12-plus-hour fast	Coffee or tea
MCT oil	Vinegar
Red wine	Turmeric
Goat cheese	Plunges in ice-cold water
Dietary fiber	Hot saunas

Soybeans   Selenium

Vitamin D   Exposure to red light

Vitamin K$_2$

You've likely already guessed the answer. All these items make, or are themselves, signaling molecules that instruct your mitochondria to uncouple. Ketones tell your mitochondria to go into repair mode and keep themselves healthy and functional—as do red wine and infrared light. All these very different influences and substances can activate mitochondrial uncoupling.

We've spent far too long arguing that ketones are an efficient super fuel that helps us burn fat. That's not the case. Ironically, Drs. Owens and Cahill, the very fathers of modern ketone theory, proved as much decades ago. What is now apparent is that ketones are, first and foremost, signaling molecules, providing critical messages to your mitochondria about what to do and when to do it. This signaling is very important. Because when mitochondria are overworked or stressed, they can be damaged by ROSs. By sending all these messages, ketones can help (a) stop the damage from occurring, (b) initiate repair of any existing damage, and (c) make more mitochondria to help carry the load.

Simply stated, we now understand you can harness all the advantages of keto, achieving weight loss and improved health, by promoting mitochondrial uncoupling, mitogenesis, and mitochondrial repair. All the benefits of a restrictive low-carb, high-fat diet, with none of the hassle (and less unappetizing fat)! Truly, mitochondrial uncoupling is the key that can help you finally crack the keto code.

Unlocking Antiaging

Most of the theories about the ways the body declines with age center on the idea of mitochondrial damage—that after decades upon decades of making ATP, your mitochondria eventually become damaged enough that they either retire or, worse, cause the cell they are living in to literally explode, a biological process known as apoptosis. But what if there was a way to hack aging by helping your mitochondria to live better, longer?

Every single mitochondrion in your body contains a coenzyme called nicotinamide adenine dinucleotide (NAD+). Simply explained, using baseball terminology, NAD+ acts as the second baseman in a double play within your electron transport chain. Imagine a baseball game where you have a player on first base. When the next player hits the ball (which represents an electron), the shortstop catches it and immediately throws the ball to the second baseman so he can tag the first player out. Fast as lightning, he then throws it to the first baseman, grabbing that second out for the team. This molecular second baseman (NAD+) is the linchpin in this double play, moving the electron ball around the bases rapidly. In mitochondria, there are no outs, of course—but all that electron movement helps make more energy. That's likely why multiple studies have shown that the more NAD+ you have in your mitochondria, the longer you'll live. Like with baseball, the better your second baseman, the more double plays you can make, and the more wins your team will rack up. At the end of the day, healthy aging comes down to those kinds of wins. And yet as we age, levels of NAD+ decline.

Ketones are known to preserve vital NAD+ molecules. My good friend Dr. David Sinclair, codirector of the Paul F. Glenn Center for Biology of Aging at Harvard Medical School, has helped uncover the fundamental role NAD+ plays in our metabolism.[8] His work has shown that ketones, as well as resveratrol (a polyphenol found in foods ranging from pistachios to red wine), can activate a special family of genes called sirtuin genes. These genes are metabolic regulators and help protect our mitochondria from damage by—you guessed it—uncoupling mitochondria, among other actions. In doing so, they also help preserve our NAD+ stores. So not only do polyphenols and ketones uncouple mitochondria—they also promote longevity and help our bodies retain NAD+ by turning on sirtuin genes.[9]

But I'm not done. Postbiotics—those signaling molecules produced in your gut—can also preserve NAD+ and uncouple mitochondria.[10] Honestly, anything that stimulates your gut bacteria to make short-chain fatty acids (SCFAs) like butyrate and acetate, whether through the consumption of fiber, fermented foods, or polyphenol-rich fare, has the power to uncouple mitochondria via SCFA production. They, in turn, also signal those sirtuin genes to get to work.

Fun fact: Studies have shown that so-called super agers—people who live to an extremely old age while managing to avoid common diseases of aging—have a lot of uncoupled mitochondria![11]

Are you sensing a pattern here? As I said before, the power of mitochondrial uncoupling has been hiding in plain sight for some time. It's just taken us some time to put all the pieces of the puzzle together. It's a good thing, too, as it means there is an array of different tools we can use to help promote good health across the life-span.

CHAPTER 5

THE KEYS THAT UNLOCK THE KETO CODE

Many keto devotees (and I was not one of them) will tell you that the effects of the diet are wholly driven by severely restricting your carb intake. Yet, a look at the foods allowed on my Keto Intensive Care Program in *The Plant Paradox* shows a lot of interesting carbs and a ton of polypehenols! I knew from twenty-plus years of patient experience that my keto program that still had lots of carbs worked, yet I didn't know quite how it worked so well. But, having learned more about the power of mitochondrial uncoupling, I now know there are a variety of compounds that can signal to those mighty cellular powerhouses and let them know it's time to uncouple and thrive, and I had already recommended most of them! What's more, those keys are not limited to your diet. So what are the most powerful mechanisms to help your body unlock the reparative and calorie-wasting features of your cellular energy factories? The truth is, if you're someone who tracks the latest wellness trends, some of these interventions may already be familiar to you. In fact, many of them have long been known to benefit health. But what we didn't understand—until now—was *how* or *why* they supported our health. Ladies and gentlemen, allow me to hand you the keys that will unlock the life-enhancing power of your mitochondria.

KEY #1: INTERMITTENT FASTING OR TIME-CONTROLLED EATING

There are articles and books aplenty that suggest fasting—or abstaining from food for a certain period of time—is a miracle cure for just about any ailment. Many of these same resources also suggest that the longer you can fast, the better off you are. Yet we now understand that extensive fasting comes with a lot of downsides, ranging from decreased energy levels to the release of heavy metals and other toxins from fat cells to muscle deterioration. Though fasting for long periods of time can be detrimental, going a day or two without food is unlikely to harm healthy individuals. In fact, there is considerable merit to fasting, at least in the short term, but most experts' interpretations of how to go about it—and why you should—have missed the mark.

On the other hand, the research on calorie restriction is clear: many studies have shown that reducing the number of daily calories consumed by 25 to 30 percent can extend an animal's health span (meaning the amount of time they live disease free) as well as their life-span (how long they live). This is true for all kinds of living organisms: studies of yeasts, fruit flies, and rats have all reached the same conclusion. But for decades, scientists couldn't explain *why* caloric restriction was so beneficial to health.

Starting in the 1980s, two famous studies using rhesus monkeys, our primate cousins, went head-to-head to get to the bottom of how caloric restriction worked its magic. The first was conducted by the National Institute on Aging (NIA), the aging research arm of the

NIH.[1] The second was led by researchers at the University of Wisconsin.[2] Both studies spanned more than thirty years, comparing the health spans and life-spans of two groups of monkeys with slightly different diets.

At each institution, the researchers put one group of monkeys on a calorie-restricted diet—to the tune of a 30 percent reduction in calories. The second group was a control group; this group's food was not restricted. As expected, the animals who were calorie-restricted had vastly improved health spans, but only one group (at the University of Wisconsin) had increased longevity compared to the controls. Why did only one group of calorie-restricted monkeys live longer than the others?

When the study results were published in 2012, I, as well as many other researchers, hypothesized that though both groups of calorie-restricted monkeys were given the same number of calories, the source of those calories accounted for the different outcomes. The UW monkeys were given a relatively high-sucrose (half glucose and half fructose—better known as good ol' table sugar) and high-fat feed. The NIA group, however, was given a diet composed of more fiber and protein, not to mention lower sugar and fat. (Just to be clear, regardless of diet makeup, both groups of monkeys received 60 percent of their calories from carbs.) Since only the UW animals exhibited increased longevity, I argued that their extended life-span may be the result of the lower protein content in their feed. Researchers David Raubenheimer and Stephen Simpson from the University of Sydney made the same argument in their book, *Eat Like the Animals*. Others, however, offered different interpretations of the data. Some suggested the longevity effects could be attributed to age differences in the animals (the NIA animals were, on the whole, quite a bit younger than the UW animals when the experiment began). Others postulated that the longevity of the

UW monkeys could be chalked up to the more processed nature of their food, as the UW monkeys ate food that was "purified"—meaning it used more refined ingredients with little to no preservatives or nonnutritional chemical additives—and the NIA group did not.

Enter NIH scientist Dr. Rafael de Cabo, who was determined get to the bottom of calorie restriction and longevity once and for all.[3] He had a notion that calorie restriction alone was not responsible for the monkeys' enhanced longevity, but rather *time of eating* restriction. To test the idea, de Cabo took approximately 300 mice (292, to be exact) and separated them into six groups. Three of those groups were given the UW diet—high sucrose, higher fat, and lower protein. The other three got the NIA-style feed. He then varied *when* each group of mice ate.

Pay attention to this—it's important: Two groups of mice had access to their food 24 hours a day. They could nosh whenever they were so inclined—one group on the UW food, and the other group on the NIA grub. The next two groups were calorie restricted—that 30 percent restriction again—and were only permitted to eat once a day at three p.m. They had a much shorter eating window. The final two groups got the full number of calories like the first two groups, but they also were restricted to that single three p.m. chow time.

Can you guess what de Cabo discovered?

The groups with 24-hour food access nibbled all day and all night, whenever the mood struck. The calorie-restricted group, however, ate their food in a hurry. It's not surprising; if you got 30 percent less food every day, and it arrived all at once as a daily ration, you would probably gobble it up very quickly. True to form, the calorie-restricted animals went to town during mealtime—and the animals who were given the UW food (the high-sucrose and higher-fat feed) ate the quickest, finishing up their rations within an hour.

Meanwhile, the last two groups of animals, the time-restricted mice, finished their food in about 12 hours, and then fasted for the rest of the day. Which, for the record, is a long time for a mouse to go without a meal.

And which group of animals showed better health and longevity? Well, only four of the six groups offered evidence of metabolic flexibility, meaning their mitochondria could switch from burning glucose to burning fatty acids on a dime, and it wasn't the all-day-eating groups. It was the calorie-restricted and time-restricted groups whose diet schedule dictated a long fasting period.

Here's the first shock: it didn't matter whether the mice got the UW food or the NIA food. (Are you paying attention, keto fans?) Nor did it matter whether they were calorie-restricted or got the full number of daily calories. All that mattered was that the *eating window was condensed*. Those animals thus had mitochondria that could easily switch between fuels, helping to promote overall health and well-being.

When it came to longevity, de Cabo saw a similar trend. The calorie-restricted mice lived nearly 30 percent longer than the 24-hour eaters. No surprise there. Yet once again, the makeup of their diets made no difference at all. And the time-restricted mice? They lived 11 percent longer than the all-day snackers. Additionally, the brains and bodies of the time-restricted mice showed less beta-amyloid, the plaque-y protein associated with Alzheimer's disease and dementia.

You may be thinking, "Okay, time to drop my caloric intake by 30 percent so I can live forever!" But consider that the calorie-restricted mice ate their meager allotment of food rapidly and fasted for most of the day. The time-restricted mice got all those nice, juicy calories over a longer period but still had lengthy fasting periods.

An 11 percent increase in longevity isn't a bad outcome. In human terms, that would likely translate into living well for an additional ten years. So remember this: de Cabo discovered that the time period during which the animals were *not* eating was more important to health than the composition of their diet.

Of course, humans are not mice—but the same effects have been documented in research on humans. In a recent Italian study, researchers found that a regimen of time-restricted eating—particularly when combined with regular exercise—resulted in many of the same health-related benefits as those documented in the de Cabo study.[4]

The researchers recruited two groups of healthy athletes to participate in this study. Both groups were given the same number of total daily calories. One group ate on a regular schedule: three meals at eight a.m., one p.m., and eight p.m. This amounted to a 12-hour eating window. The second group ate the same three meals within a 7-hour window, with mealtimes at one p.m., four p.m., and finishing the last meal by eight p.m. The athletes who ate within the time-restricted window not only experienced fat loss and muscle mass growth, but the researchers also measured a decline in their hormone called insulin-like growth factor (IGF-1), which is known to drive the aging process. The 12-hour eaters did not experience any of these benefits, despite eating the *exact same number of calories*. Same calories, different results. So much for the "calories in, calories out" theory of weight loss!

The question then became, what is the secret to time-controlled eating? Here's where our ketone friends come into play. Having a longer fasting window compels the liver to produce more ketones, which in turn signal the mitochondria to become more resilient, stronger, and healthier—by wasting fuel, multiplying, and repairing themselves by uncoupling. The more you compress that eating window, the longer your mitochondria will be exposed to ketones and the effects of mitochondrial uncoupling—and the more health benefits you will reap. The news flash here is that you don't need to eat a diet of 80 percent fat to lose weight and boost your health span and longevity.

Glucose stores (glycogen) last for about 12 hours. It's at that point or thereabouts that our bodies start liberating fatty acids from our fat stores—some of which head to the liver to be converted into ketones. If you have normal insulin levels (unfortunately, most Americans do not), it is normal, within the course of a 24-hour day, to cycle in and out of ketosis, burning sugar (glucose) as fuel and then, after a 12-hour fasting window, making ketones, which do not provide a new type of super fuel, as we once thought, but instead signal that it's time to uncouple mitochondria.[5]

The big idea here is not that fasting has positive health effects— we've known that for millennia. Rather, what I hope you take away is that it's not *what* you eat that matters the most to a healthy metabolism, but *when* and for *how long* you eat. That's why I recommend that my patients try to maintain a fasting window of at least 16 hours. That gives your body enough time to not only use up glycogen, but free up those FFAs and start making those miraculous mitochondrial signalers: ketones.

One last proviso before you decide to eat an entire chocolate cake as your only meal of the day. Obviously, all the mice in de Cabo's study eventually died, but fascinatingly, the mice who ate the high-sucrose, high-fat UW diet were more likely to die of liver cancer than any other cause. While the large-scale benefits come from a condensed eating window, you are still better off filling it with healthy, whole foods, which will add additional uncoupling benefits to those you experience by restricting your eating window.

KEY #2: POLYPHENOLS

Remember how I asked you to note that "2,4-dinitrophenol" (or DNP, that miraculous weight loss drug of the 1930s and '40s) contains the word *phenol*? There's a reason, and here it is: many health experts will be quick to tell you that polyphenols (lots of phenols), the special micronutrient compounds concentrated in plant leaves, fruits, and seeds, provide antiaging effects by protecting your cells from oxidation.[6] You may have also heard that they can encourage blood vessels to remain flexible, keeping your blood pressure in a healthy range and reducing inflammation. There are also a whole host of stories about how polyphenols control blood sugar levels and modulate insulin release.[7] I haven't even gotten to the claims that polyphenols protect against cancer, Alzheimer's, cognitive decline, and neurological inflammation—or that they prevent damage to cells.[8] That's quite a list, no?

Believe it or not, the tales are all true. And I've published multiple human studies testifying to these effects. Polyphenols really do offer all these seemingly magical benefits. But they don't have a thing to do with antioxidants. Instead, these effects are the result of polyphenols uncoupling your mitochondria.[9]

Polyphenols can be found far and wide throughout the plant kingdom. They are concentrated in foods ranging from coffee and tea to cacao, berries, pomegranates, dark-colored grapes, spinach, kale, red cabbage, grains, and many medicinal herbs and spices. Basically, any dark or brightly colored plant-based food is likely to be chock-full of polyphenols (I've included a list of common sources on page 131). Several popular supplements, including grapeseed extract and Pycnogenol (maritime pine bark extract), also contain polyphenols.

Plants use polyphenols to protect their chloroplasts, the plant version of mitochondria, from damage, particularly from sunlight.

Notice the parallels here: Plants need sunlight in order for their chloroplasts to produce energy. Human mitochondria need oxygen for the same purpose. And yet both sunlight and oxygen are damaging to these organelles.[10] How do plants mitigate this damage? Ten points if you said uncoupling, brought about by the actions of their polyphenols!

Despite all the great health benefits linked to polyphenols, most of these compounds are not readily bioavailable, or easily used by the body when you ingest them. Your small intestine can only absorb about 10 percent of any polyphenol nutrients you consume. But unabsorbed polyphenols have their own benefits: they act as prebiotics in the gut, feeding the beneficial microbes that promote good health. Your gut buddies gobble up these compounds and convert them into forms that are more absorbable. In the process, they also create postbiotics—the signaling molecules that unlock your mitochondria.[11]

Most plant-based foods contain more than one type of polyphenol. In fact, scientists have now identified literally thousands of different compounds that fall into this category, which have been further subdivided into four main groups: flavonoids, phenolic acids, lignans, and stilbenes. Flavonoids, the brightly colored plant pigments like quercetin, anthocyanins, kaempferol, and catechins, are found in foods like onions, dark chocolate, and red cabbage, to name just a few. Phenolic acids and stilbenes are found in many fruits and veggies. Lignans are found in seeds like flaxseeds and sesame seeds. Raspberries contain a different polyphenol called ellagic acid, while the turmeric in your spice cabinet gets its vivid color from curcumin. The type of polyphenol, as well as the amount, varies from food to food—and may also change based on where the plant grows, its ripeness, and how it is prepared. Regardless, the more polyphenols you consume, the better.

It bears mentioning that olives and olive oil are considered such great health foods not just because of the monounsaturated fat (oleic acid) they contain, but because they're chock-full of polyphenols that—you guessed it—tell mitochondria to uncouple. For example, hydroxytyrosol (HT), one of those polyphenols, is considered one of the key factors responsible for the Mediterranean diet's many health benefits. Research using olive oil extract has shown that HT likely prevents cardiovascular disease and other diseases of aging by stimulating mitogenesis—which, if you recall, is exactly what uncoupling mitochondria achieves.[12]

I'd be remiss if I didn't mention one more thing about polyphenols. Have you ever noticed that a cup of coffee or tea, even an iced variety, can make you feel flushed? Surprise! Polyphenols, as well as the caffeine in these drinks, uncouple your mitochondria, which in turn produces heat.[13] What about the feelings of heat you experience after a glass of red wine, an ice-cold beer, or a margarita? The polyphenols in these alcoholic drinks, as well as the alcohol itself, are uncouplers.[14]

Tricolor Fat: White, Brown, and Beige

Given all this discussion of uncouplers, it's worth taking a closer look at your adipose tissue, or body fat. Adipose tissue is classified primarily as either brown adipose tissue (BAT) or white adipose tissue (WAT). The latter stores the majority of our excess calories. BAT, however, which we talked a bit about earlier, is responsible for a process called nonshivering thermogenesis, which helps produce heat.

Long ago, I was taught that we had BAT to enable babies and

small mammals to produce heat by burning more calories, rather than shivering to produce heat, in order to better adapt to colder temperatures. In fact, a few decades ago, most researchers would have told you that brown fat mysteriously disappears as you grow into adulthood. Ten years ago, however, my colleagues made an amazing discovery: adult humans retain deposits of brown fat, mostly below the neck and around the collarbones. Furthermore, that brown fat is metabolically active, packed to the gills with mitochondria. White fat, in comparison, doesn't normally contain a lot of mitochondria.

You probably know where I'm going with this. Brown fat generates heat because it burns more calories than white fat. Or should I say *wastes* more calories? Yes, here again, the mitochondria in brown fat uncouple and generate heat in the process.

While much of the discussion about fat in the nutrition and health fields concerns the white and brown varieties, there is a third type of fat: beige fat. Essentially, this is white fat that is starting to transform into brown fat—hence the "beige" designation. Studies have shown that the more beige fat cells you have, the lower your body mass index (BMI) will be. How does this fat get its signature color and lead to that healthier weight? You already know what I'm going to say. It has more mitochondria. Mitochondria that can uncouple!

Fun fact: Polyphenols can help convert your white fat to beige fat. Compounds like curcumin, found in the bright yellow spice turmeric,[15] as well as berberine,[16] a polyphenol you can find in Oregon grape root, barberry, and goldenseal, can help transform white fat into brown and beige fat.

The amount of brown fat in your body can tell a doctor a lot about your health status; I already mentioned BMI. In a study of 52,000 patients at the Memorial Sloan Kettering Cancer Center, researchers discovered that patients with the most BAT were the healthiest overall.[17] For example, only 4.6 percent of patients with the most BAT had type 2 diabetes, as opposed to 9 percent of those with the least BAT. People with brown fat also tend to have a lower risk of developing hypertension, congestive heart failure, and coronary heart disease, and it's thought to mitigate the negative health effects of obesity. In fact, research shows that, generally speaking, overweight people with the most brown fat appeared as healthy as those who were not overweight or obese.

Not all body fat is created equal—and eating a diet rich in polyphenols can help you convert your white fat to the beige and brown varieties, supporting more mitochondrial uncoupling and, by extension, better health and well-being.

KEY #3: DIETARY FIBER

Polyphenols aren't the only reason plant-based foods are so important to health and longevity. Most of those foods are also chock-full of dietary fiber.

Remember, your gut buddies need good nutrition to make their valuable postbiotics. And what do they most love to eat? Fibrous plant-based foods! When our gut bacteria consume their favorite prebiotic foods, they ferment them to create postbiotic signaling compounds such as acetate and butyrate. They also make signaling compounds in the form of gasses, called gasotransmitters, like hydrogen and hydrogen sulfide and nitric oxide.

Our hunter-gatherer ancestors consumed about 150 grams of fiber *each day*. That's a lot of leaves, tubers, and seeds! Compare that number to the measly 5 grams a day we consume in the typical modern American diet.[18] Even those of us who consume a lot of plant-based foods would find it a challenge to top 60 grams of fiber. And if you're on a traditional ketogenic diet, you may not manage even a single gram. This lack of fiber intake, unfortunately, is strongly associated with poor health.[19] Conversely, studies suggest that the more fiber you eat, the healthier you are.

That doesn't mean you should run out and buy some high-fiber cereal or start sprinkling wheat bran on everything. Most of the fiber found in whole grains (as well as some plants) is accompanied by lectins—proteins that can harm gut health and generate widespread inflammation. Your gut buddies are most partial to soluble fibers (those that dissolve in water) like inulin, found in multiple plant foods, which they can gobble up to make butyrate and other postbiotics.

Interestingly, butyrate is not only a mitochondrial uncoupler; it is also used as a building block for the ketone called beta-hydroxybutyrate (BHB). Acetate or acetic acid (you may know it as vinegar), another postbiotic, is also used by the body to make ketones and is a mitochondrial uncoupler by itself.[20] It really does come full circle: butyrate and acetate tell your mitochondria to waste fuel, create more of themselves, and take the time to make necessary repairs. No matter which way you get there, mitochondrial uncoupling is the key.

Fiber for Longevity

Swedish researcher Dr. Staffan Lindeberg spent his career studying the Kitavan people, a group of about two thousand Indigenous people who inhabit the South Pacific island of Kitava, which is part of Papua New Guinea. The Kitavans are traditional farmers who consume a significant quantity of fibrous vegetables. Their high-fiber diet includes tubers like yam, sweet potato, and taro (all lectin-free, I might add!), as well local fishes, fresh fruits, and coconut. In fact, about 60 percent of their daily calories come from coconuts (to be clear here, coconuts, not coconut oil).

Lindeberg discovered something fascinating about the Kitavans: they live longer than their Western counterparts and enjoy a better health span, free of most of the cardiovascular diseases that plague industrialized societies. (And that's despite smoking like fiends—but we'll talk more about nicotine and its role in mitochondrial uncoupling later.)

It also bears mentioning that the Kitavans are generally quite thin, despite eating a lot of food—their daily caloric intake is significant.[21] How do they stay so trim? I suspect all the prebiotic fiber they consume is feeding their gut microbes, which are making plenty of butyrate from all that fiber. They probably also get a ketone boost from the MCTs in coconuts. Between the ketones and the fiber, their mitochondria get plenty of messages to waste calories, multiply, and take good care of themselves and their Kitavan hosts.

KEY #4: FERMENTED FOODS

I'm not the first person to tout the health benefits of fermented foods like vinegar, yogurt, sauerkraut, aged cheese, wine, and miso. But I may be the first to suggest that these foods don't work their wonders just by being a great source of probiotics, the bacteria that populate the microbiome. In fact, while some of these foods contain some living bacteria, most living microbes are destroyed by cooking and preparation processes before you eat them. Also, even if you did eat these foods raw, the probiotics likely wouldn't make it past the acids in your stomach to reach your colon.

Why might fermented foods be so good for you, then? Well, when you eat these foods, you're consuming the products of fermentation naturally within them, including short-chain fatty acids like acetate, butyrate, propionate, and malic acid. The fermentation process can also make medium-chain fatty acids, MCTs. All these by-products are mitochondrial uncouplers. Imagine: a splash of apple cider vinegar, a glass of your favorite wine, and some finely aged cheese all produce their health benefits via the same mechanisms. Fermentation by-products that promote mitochondrial uncoupling are the key.[22] Indeed, a recent paper from researchers at Stanford University shows that fermented foods dramatically improve microbiome diversity and suppress inflammation in humans—and do so more than eating a high-fiber diet.[23] I propose such a finding proves that you can get an added "pop" from the mitochondrial uncouplers in fermented foods.

Melatonin Handles the Night Shift

You likely know that the hormone melatonin plays an important role in our sleep-wake cycle. Your doctor may have even suggested that you take a melatonin supplement before bed to help you fall asleep. But as you'll learn later in this book, melatonin isn't the "sleep hormone." Rather, its real work starts when you're already asleep. Not only does it work as a bouncer at the Mito Club; melatonin is also yet another key that unlocks our mitochondria, telling them to uncouple and repair themselves while we sleep.[24]

KEY #5: POLYAMINES

Polyphenols aren't the only food-based compounds that can unlock health benefits. Polyamines, organic compounds found in foods like aged cheeses and mushrooms, can uncouple mitochondria as well.[25] In fact, numerous studies support the idea that polyamines play a significant role in longevity. In one such study, rodents that consumed polyamines lived 25 percent longer than control animals that did not.[26] Other studies have shown polyamine consumption can protect against heart disease and age-related memory loss.[27] In studies of long-lived individuals, researchers have found that centenarians, people who live to the ripe old age of one hundred or beyond, have high levels of these compounds in their blood and tissues.[28]

Polyamines may also play a role in the so-called French paradox. As you may know, the French consume a lot of saturated fat. How could they not—that cheese is divine! Yet despite their propensity for high-fat eating, they have a relatively low incidence of heart disease—and, correspondingly, a low rate of death from such conditions. Some in the medical community have chalked up this phenomenon to the fact that the French wash down all that saturated fat with red wine, which contains the polyphenols resveratrol, quercetin, and melatonin. While resveratrol may contribute to the French paradox, I suspect there's another factor at play: the regular consumption of aged cow's-, goat's-, and sheep's-milk cheeses—all rich in polyamines. Goat's- and sheep's-milk cheeses are also an impressive source of MCTs, which, as you know, boost mitochondrial health by being converted into ketones.

You can find polyamines in nuts and seeds, shellfish, soybeans, and tea leaves.[29] And in fermented foods, including miso, natto, and soy sauce, the fermentation process produces the polyamines putrescine and histamine.

Harness the Power of Plant Energy

Let's pause a moment to review why uncoupling proteins exist across both plant and animal species. (If you recall, humans have five of these vital proteins.) The concepts are important and will help you understand why the recommendations in the Keto Code plan are so effective.

Plants rely on sunlight for energy. The energy factories of their cells are not mitochondria but chloroplasts, which use light to convert water and carbon dioxide into oxygen, glucose, and ATP. Sunlight is essential for making ATP, but it can damage chloroplasts in the same way that oxygen, generally necessary for ATP production in animals, can ravage mitochondria. Truly, here is a situation where you can't live with it, can't live without it. But both plant and animal cells have a built-in buffering system to help mitigate the harms that come from energy production: In plants, this buffering system consists of polyphenols and melatonin.

When plants are under stress caused by heat, drought, or high elevation (which places them closer to the sun), they activate more uncoupling in their chloroplasts to protect themselves.[30] That creates a cycle: The greater the stress, the greater the production of polyphenols and melatonin. The greater the production of polyphenols and melatonin, the greater the mitochondrial uncoupling—and with it, more mitochondrial protection, repair, and multiplication.

When we eat plants rich in polyphenols and melatonin, these compounds send the same uncoupling messages to our own mitochondria, whether or not ketones or postbiotics are present. Our health, weight, and longevity all benefit as a result. In fact, one reason I recommend organic fruits and vegetables is that growing under far more nutrient and pest stress than conventional produce means they have a much higher polyphenol content.[31]

KEY #6: COLD TEMPERATURES

You likely noticed the first six keys are all food-related; how could a change in temperature impact your health? Cold-water plunges or cold showers—a practice that has become popular in recent years thanks to evangelizers like Wim Hof, as well as a host of other health experts—also result in the production of a protein that helps regulate metabolism and, no surprise by now, is a mitochondrial uncoupler.[32]

It appears that all those Scandinavians who take cold-water plunges have been onto something for centuries. But you don't have to join your local Polar Bear Club to harness the uncoupling potential of cold. Instead, you can start your day with a "Scottish shower": Take your usual warm shower. Once you've finished washing, slowly reduce the hot water flow until the water runs cold. Now comes the more difficult part. Once the water is as cold as you can get it, remain under the stream for a full minute. It will definitely wake you up! And it will also leave you and your mitochondria feeling invigorated. (For those who think this option is too extreme, you can also try a cold vest, a product that wraps your shoulders and upper chest in removable ice packs with the goal of converting your white fat to healthy beige fat.)

If even thinking about the cold immediately brings on the shivers, understand that your body has a greater capacity to handle cold water than you might think—which is why I recommend the cold shower approach to my patients. Starting out with just ten seconds and then gradually increasing your time under the shower's chilly spray will not only help you adjust your mind-set, but will increase your body's tolerance to the cold.

KEY #7: HOT TEMPERATURES

On the other end of the temperature spectrum, heat can also unlock mitochondria. Like dogs, cats, horses, and all other mammals (as well as a few fish), we are endotherms, warm-blooded animals capable of generating our own heat. Our mitochondria act as tiny radiators, creating most of the heat in our bodies. And we need it— the brain is put at risk when glucose and oxygen are in short supply. The mitochondria of warm-blooded animals, luckily, run at a higher temperature than the body's normal 97 to 99°F.[33] It's even been suggested that mitochondria function optimally at a steamy 122°F— an incredible 25 degrees hotter than typical body temperature![34]

Recent studies have also shown that the activation of uncoupling proteins in neurons, especially those located in regions like the hypothalamus (the part of the brain that regulates energy maintenance) and the hippocampus (the brain's memory center), increase local heat in those cells. What's more, the neurons appreciate that increase in temperature, as it improves their individual function while simultaneously prompting a slight decrease in overall body temperature.[35] I told you I'd come back to thermogenesis—but we'll dive deeper into this phenomenon in chapter 9.

KEY #8: RED LIGHT THERAPY

In recent years, clinicians have relied on near-infrared light therapy to help treat both ophthalmological and neurological issues. The intervention is based on the assumption that this frequency of light can improve mitochondrial function. But might its benefits also be the result of heat production?

Scientists have observed that individuals who experience hyperthermia, or people who are otherwise healthy but have a body temperature that runs a little higher than normal, have brains that work more efficiently. It's possible that these high temperatures help optimize neural signaling, which would be a good thing for a person with epilepsy—epileptic seizures are the result of neurons becoming overly excited and firing off willy-nilly. As I've said before, ketones probably weren't successful in reducing seizures because of their reputation as a super fuel. It's more likely that by signaling mitochondria to uncouple, the temperature of neurons rose and the excitability of those cells dropped. Too much warming can harm the brain, no doubt—but a little heat every now and again can be quite beneficial even to people who have not been diagnosed with a seizure disorder.

While they do not emit heat, red and near-infrared light can also work directly on mitochondria. Typically, the parts of our eyes that take in light have the highest mitochondrial density. That's one reason our retinas age so much faster than our other organs do—you may start to see some decline in your vision in your forties. Researchers have found that short bursts of red light in longer wavelengths can reverse some of these age-related effects, rebooting the retina's cells in just a few minutes a day.[36]

What might account for such an improvement? Certain spectrums of red light signal mitochondria to uncouple. In fact, these treatments are so successful that red light therapy has been approved by the FDA as an antiaging therapy (as well as for pain relief, wound healing, and other health issues).[37]

There you have it: the keys to unlocking the keto code! It's amazing, isn't it? All these diverse and seemingly unrelated foods, dietary practices, and other interventions converge at the same endpoint: to help support your mitochondria and ensure they are working at their full potential. You no longer have to suffer through fat-centric meals. You don't have to worry about not finding something you can enjoy when out at a restaurant with your family or friends. And you don't have to give up your favorite plant-based foods in a futile attempt to reach "ketosis." By embracing these eight keys, you can leverage all the benefits of keto without the hassle, boredom, or associated health risks. Talk about a win-win situation!

CHAPTER 6

THE TRUTH ABOUT FATS

Chances are, you've been given a lot of bad information about fat. For decades, health experts recommended fats be avoided at all costs—with no differentiation between the various types of fat. More recently, as keto diets have emerged as a leading health trend, that advice has changed—and quite dramatically! Suddenly, you can't eat too much fat—no matter what kind. You supposedly need it to make the ketones that so-called keto experts suggest are your body's preferred fuel source. Not!

Today we know that some fats offer health benefits, but the guidance peddled by many keto programs—that all fats should be eaten with abandon—couldn't be further from the truth. In fact, there are many different kinds of fats (more than you may even be familiar with!) and each of them plays a different role in the body. In order to understand which fats best support health and weight loss, it's important to learn a little bit more about their chemistry.

Scientifically speaking, fats are categorized by how many sets of fatty acids (which are carbon atoms) are attached lengthwise along a backbone of sugar (glycerol). At your last annual physical, your doctor likely shared your triglyceride number from your cholesterol test. This number is the easiest way to understand how many sugars and starches you've been converting into storable fat. Yes, your body converts any extra sugar (carbs), especially the sugar in fruit, into fat!

Depending on how many fatty acids are linked in a row, fats are classified as very-long-, long-, medium-, or short-chain fatty acids. We've already talked about some of the short-chain fatty acids (SCFAs) in previous chapters. Postbiotics like acetate, butyrate, and propionate are all SCFAs.

Then you've got your medium-chain fatty acids, also referred to as medium-chain triglycerides (MCTs). This group of fatty acids includes valeric acid, as well as caproic, caprylic, and capric acids. The names of these fats are derived from *capra*, the Latin word for the genus of goat, because the latter three are found in abundance in goat's milk. And when it comes to unlocking the keto code, MCTs truly are the GOAT of all fats! (Coconut oil contains another MCT called lauric acid, but despite all the recent fanfare about coconut oil, it actually has little to no ketogenic potential.)

Fats with thirteen or more carbon atoms are long-chain fatty acids (LCFAs). These are the fats found in dairy products, vegetable and seed oils, and olive oil. And if your fat chain has more than twenty-two carbon atoms? Those are very-long-chain fatty acids (VLCFAs). The latest studies suggest these fats may play important roles in neural function—we'll get into more detail about their role in cognitive health shortly.

You can think of triglycerides as the means of transportation for fats. These chains, composed of three glycerols and their attached fatty acids (hence the name *triglyceride*), allow fats to get to where they need to go. When fatty acids are incorporated into triglycerides, becoming part of the chain, they can be moved to and from storage in fat cells. They are also, minus the glycerol backbone, a key component of the membranes that surround every cell in your body and, as luck would have it, the inner and outer membranes of the mitochondria.

Most of the fats we consume contain more than one type of fatty acid chain, but they tend to be characterized by the predominant one. With that in mind, let's take a closer look at the various types of fat you eat every day and the role each plays in your health and well-being.

Short-chain fatty acids (SFCAs). SCFAs are the superstars of the postbiotic world. Butyrate, for example, contributes to somewhere in the vicinity of 10 percent of your system-wide energy production, playing an especially vital role in ensuring your gut has enough energy to function. Butyrate is also the primary fuel source for your colon,[1] where it helps keep this organ's cells healthy and happy (and helps prevent cancers from forming).[2] Additionally, butyrate handles communication between the microbiome and the immune system, sending messages that drive the production of important hormones to keep inflammation at bay across the body.

Butyrate that isn't being used by the gut can travel through your lymphatic system and bloodstream, delivering important information to your cells. That's how it ultimately reaches your mitochondria to let them know it's time to uncouple. In order to reap the benefits of these compounds, you need to eat plenty of soluble plant fiber, which feeds your gut buddies the foods they love so they then make postbiotics. Fermented foods, wine, vinegar, and aged cheeses are also good sources of preformed SCFAs.

Medium-chain triglycerides (MCTs). MCTs are a fascinating type of fat—they are instantly absorbed without the aid of digestive enzymes. And unlike all other fats, they don't need special molecules to ferry them across the gut wall. This kind of accessibility means that MCTs can go directly to the liver, where they're converted into ketones—regardless of your carb and protein intake. If you have adequate MCTs in your diet, you can generate the same amount of ketones as you would by fasting or eating in the traditional keto fashion. This is why MCTs truly are the GOAT of this program! When you ingest MCTs, you don't need to get 80 percent of your calories from fat. Instead, you can fill your plate with delicious plant-based foods and still harness all the power of mitochondrial uncoupling.

MCTs are available as MCT oil and MCT powder, and constitute 30 percent of the fats in goat, sheep, and water buffalo milk products such as yogurts, kefirs, and cheeses. They are a delicious addition to the Keto Code program!

I've long championed MCT oil, but I have to admit that until recently, I didn't fully understand why it had such profound health benefits, besides being converted directly into ketones. In a landmark 2008 study, researchers from Columbia University compared two groups of overweight people eating a diet with the same number of daily calories with one critical difference: one group ate olive oil—the superfood credited with most of the Mediterranean diet's success—while the other group consumed MCT oil. Fascinatingly, the individuals who ate MCT oil generated more heat, burned more oxygen, and lost more weight than those who consumed olive oil.[3] Let me repeat that: the amount of weight lost *was not determined by caloric intake* but rather by the type of oil they consumed. In another study, researchers compared the use of MCT oil and olive oil in an otherwise similar weight loss program. The people in the MCT oil group lost an average of 3.7 pounds more than those in the olive oil group.[4] To continue our Mito Club metaphor, the MCT oil group was able to waste calories by letting them out through their emergency exits!

Long-chain fatty acids (LCFAs). These fats are those we commonly refer to as saturated, monounsaturated, and polyunsaturated fats. Saturated fats include palmitic and stearic acids, like you'd find in butter, liver, and many cheeses. The monounsaturated category includes oleic acid, the predominant fat in olive oil and avocado oil. Polyunsaturated fats (PUFAs), found in most seed oils, include omega-6 fats like linoleic acid (LA) and omega-3 fats like alpha-linolenic acid (ALA). You may have heard these referred to as "essential fatty acids." And for good reason! Our cells, including our mitochondria, need them to function, but our bodies don't make them. The only way for our cells to get these essential building blocks is for us to consume them.

I should add that there are also some unsung superstar uncouplers in the polyunsaturated category: omega-7, found in macadamia nut oil and sea buckthorn oil, and omega-5, found in pomegranate seed oil and bitter melon seed oil, send all the right messages to your mitochondria.[5]

Recently, there has been quite a bit of fearmongering by some health experts about polyunsaturated fats like LA and ALA. They suggest that PUFAs are linked to debilitating medical conditions like heart disease, arthritis, and diabetes. I hate to rain on their parade, but both of these fats are essential components of your mitochondrial membranes. Indeed, ALA (present in organic canola and flaxseed oils) may be the unsung hero in reversing and preventing heart disease! I'll have more to say about how these PUFAs have been unnecessarily thrown under the bus—but we now understand they are only guilty by association, thanks to diets full of sugar—in chapter 8.

That said, if your goal is to lose weight, you want to eat LCFAs in moderation. Despite the fact that most traditional keto diets tell you to fill up on fatty meats, butter, cream cheese, and, of course, bacon, eating these foods can make it harder to lose weight. In fact, LCFAs have actually been shown to *block* weight loss—by both impairing your cells' ability to make energy and increasing insulin resistance. Studies show that LCFAs increase the production of a metabolic enzyme that *decreases* glucose metabolism.[6] It's likely why fasting glucose levels are elevated in individuals who eat a traditional high-fat ketogenic diet despite the fact that they aren't consuming many carbs.[7] Is it any wonder that my patient Miranda was holding on to extra pounds despite trying to follow the traditional keto diet to the letter?

BETTER OUTCOMES, LESS HASSLE

Once you connect all the dots, you can see weight loss is intrinsically tied to the calorie-wasting ability of your mitochondria and whether they're receiving the signal to waste energy. Normally, eating a significant amount of carbohydrates and/or overdoing it on the protein front would suppress ketone production. But this does not occur when you either consume sufficient MCT oil, increase the time window each day when you are *not* eating, or consume foods and/or polyphenols that promote uncoupling.

The great news is, the ketones generated after consuming MCTs send the same signals to our mitochondria as the ketones that come from a full-out ketogenic diet or frank starvation. But it's not a 24/7 phenomenon. In fact, it's just the opposite! And because you aren't in ketosis all the time, you don't have to suffer its unpleasant side effects, including muscle wasting and brain fog.

Simply stated, the Keto Code program offers you an easier, more effective, and healthier way to unlock the benefits of keto. And when I say easier, I mean it. You can tailor the program to suit your own dietary preferences and eat what you want. You can follow a vegan or vegetarian diet, if you like. You can avoid red meat and consume only fish and shellfish as your protein sources, or you can enjoy a wide mix of meat, poultry, and seafood dishes. There's no need to follow an exceedingly restrictive diet to make uncoupling work for you. You need only follow three simple rules.

Rule #1: Consume some of your fats in the form of MCTs.

How many MCTs should you aim for? Multiple studies have shown that 30 grams (approximately 1 tablespoon) of MCT oil is usually enough to achieve a blood ketone level high enough to produce positive effects on both brain function and metabolism.[8] MCT oil (now available in many grocery stores, even Costco, and through many online outlets) is flavorless, odorless, and remarkably easy to add to your diet, either by drinking it, mixing it in coffee or tea, or mixing it half and half with olive oil in salad dressings. On this program, we will slowly increase your MCT dose to hit that Goldilocks "just right" sweet spot. There's also a plethora of foods that contain a substantial portion of MCT fats (see chapter 10).

Another benefit to using MCT oil is that you're able to include more carbs—those fiber-rich and nutrient-dense plant-based foods—in your meals. As your liver produces ketones from MCT oil and benefits from having a chance to rest between meals (see Rule #2), you'll be able to get the results you're looking for without the gustatorial boredom that leads so many people to abandon traditional keto programs.

The Rats That Couldn't Maintain Their Weight

In a 2020 study that assessed the impact of the keto diet on exercise capacity, Japanese scientists divided a group of rats into three subgroups.[9] One group was fed conventional high-carbohydrate rodent chow, the second was given a keto diet full of LCFAs, and the third was fed a keto diet rich in MCTs.

The researchers quickly encountered an unexpected problem that illustrates the power of MCTs: the longer the rats were on the MCT-enhanced keto diet, the more weight they lost and the less hungry they became. This meant that compared to the other two rat groups, they were consuming significantly fewer calories and losing too much weight. In order to keep the study from being sabotaged by the less hungry rats, the scientists adjusted their diets. They ultimately found that the rats eating an MCT-enhanced keto diet would eat calories comparable to the number the other rats ate when the ratio of their diet was changed to 16 percent protein, 66 percent fat, and 18 percent carbohydrate. (In comparison, the LCFA keto diet, which contained the same number of calories, was made up of 12 percent protein, 87 percent fat, and 1 percent carbohydrate—that's a pretty significant difference.) In the end, only the rats on the MCT keto diet lost weight; the LCFA keto diet rats, in comparison, didn't lose any weight at all. I can think of more than a few patients who would be glad to know of this study. Even when you're doing keto "right," it can be tough to get the results you're looking for.

Rule #2: Follow a time-restricted eating plan.

We've been through this: the longer you go without eating (up to a point), the more ketones your liver will produce. On the Keto Code program, your goal will be to limit your eating to a window of 6 to 8 hours.

If that sounds intimidating, rest assured: I'll show you how to gradually build toward an eating schedule that works for you. It's not easy to shift from a glucose-driven metabolism to a fat-driven one in a 24-hour period. I'll explain how to achieve that flexibility, enabling you to generate ketones through time-controlled eating during the week and consuming MCT oil as a supplement to kickstart ketone production.

Rule #3: Feast on fermented foods and fiber.

We tend to think of fermented foods such as sauerkraut and miso paste as rich sources of gut-boosting probiotics. But these foods play another, perhaps more important role: the fermentation process produces acetate or acetic acid (vinegar), an SCFA and mitochondrial uncoupler.[10]

In addition, acetate has been shown to offer neuroprotective benefits. In a recent study using geriatric mice, researchers showed that consuming acetate ameliorated the cognitive defects that would normally occur from the trauma of surgery.[11] The acetate signaled special cells called microglia, the neurons' bodyguards, and told them not to overreact. It also sent signals to neurons to uncouple their mitochondria so they could protect themselves during surgery. (Remember this study when we discuss brain health in the next chapter.) What's important is that fermented foods don't work solely by being a rich source of probiotics, but because the fermentation process produces SCFAs, those incredible mitochondrial uncouplers.

Acetate, butyrate, propionate, and pentanoate are, as mentioned earlier, postbiotics. They are also produced by your gut bacteria when they ferment (eat) fibrous foods and resistant starches. You should know that both acetate and butyrate also prevent mitochondrial dysfunction by protecting them from the overproduction of reactive oxygen species (ROSs), those rowdy players from the Mito Club.[12] Acetate is more efficient in enhancing metabolism and inhibiting ROSs than butyrate, but butyrate can more effectively inhibit the generation of excessive nitric oxide, which can break down the mitochondria. One study even noted that SCFAs provide an easy-to-find method to reverse or prevent type 2 diabetes.[13] They do so by uncoupling mitochondria directly, sending them the molecular signal to start repairing themselves and multiply, and, in the process, waste more calories. No wonder apple cider vinegar has such a fan club.[14]

EXERCISE YOUR OPTIONS

While weight loss is the goal of many who try adopting a keto diet, other people struggle with the traditional version because they feel it negatively impacts their athletic performance and endurance. Research has shown mixed results when it comes to athletic performance on keto, but generally speaking, the diet tends to make it harder to sustain their energy levels during high-endurance activities like running and cycling.[15]

In one study, researchers found that athletes following a ketogenic diet had to consume more oxygen by breathing faster and harder in order to achieve the same level of performance as those who ate a high-carbohydrate diet. In addition, as mentioned earlier, following a ketogenic diet over the long term has been shown to increase the production of an enzyme that slows your metabolism. When your body makes a lot of this enzyme, it prevents glucose from entering cells—the very glucose you need to call upon when you're asking your muscles to go the literal extra mile. As you might expect, this impairs an athlete's capacity for high-intensity exercise.[16]

Simply stated, this leads to more insulin resistance, which likely explains why followers of the traditional ketogenic diet have such high fasting glucose levels.[17] This is not the metabolic state you want to be in to promote long-term health or support athletic performance.

CHOOSE YOUR FATS WISELY

Bottom line: There are distinctions among fats—and those differences influence your weight, health span, and life-span.[18] Truly, your health demands that you understand what sets them apart from one another. When you eat the right kinds of fats, like the SCFAs found in fermented foods or MCTs, our program GOAT (even sourced from actual goat products, if you like!), your liver will be compelled to produce ketones that will signal your mitochondria to uncouple. That, in turn, leads to the wasting of calories, as well as mitogenesis and mitochondrial repair. Eating the right fats in the right amounts, rather than the monstrous amounts of the wrong fats that so many of us eat regularly (and that are promoted in a traditional keto diet), can get you there with relative ease.

A Quick Fats Reference Guide

I realize your head may be spinning a bit from all the discussion of fats. But it's important to remember that eating the right fats can make or break you when it comes to unlocking the keto code. Here's an easy way to remember the different types of fats and what they do:

SHORT-CHAIN FATTY ACIDS (SCFAS)

Found In: Fermented foods and some types of cheese, butter, and cow's milk. These types of fats are also made by your gut bacteria when you eat foods high in fiber.

Uncoupling Power: These are direct mitochondrial uncouplers. That's why I always say, "Eat short to live long!"

MEDIUM-CHAIN TRIGLYCERIDES (MCTS)

Found In: Goat and sheep dairy products, as well as in supplement form.

Uncoupling Power: These are the fats that are immediately converted into ketones by the liver, which then uncouple mitochondria. When it comes to MCTs, you want your fats "medium well"!

LONG-CHAIN FATTY ACIDS (LCFAS)

Found In: Fatty fish like salmon and sardines, as well as meat, dairy, and eggs. You can also find different types of LCFAs in oils and nuts.

Uncoupling Power: Polyunsaturated fatty acids (PUFAs) like ALA, LA, DHA, EPA, and AA are all essential fatty acids that optimize our brain and mitochondrial function, and help promote uncoupling! Our cells, including our mitochondria, need them to work their best, but our bodies don't make them on their own—to get them, we need to consume them in foods.

You also want to try to consume the two other essential saturated fats: C15, found primarily in dairy and seafood, and C14, also from dairy. These fats are linked to improved heart health (see chapter 7). Your body can make all the rest of the saturated fats on its own; you don't need to eat them, as traditional keto doctrine suggests.

Any discussion of LCFAs needs to also mention monounsaturated fats like the oleic acid found in olive oil. I'm a huge fan of olive oil not only because it contains this fat, but because it is a carrier for polyphenols! As I like to say, "The only purpose of food is to get more olive oil into your mouth."

VERY LONG-CHAIN FATTY ACIDS (VLCFAS):

Found In: Canola oil and macadamia nuts.

Uncoupling Power: One type of VLCFA, C22, also acts as an uncoupler. And higher levels of this particular fat in the blood are associated with a reduced risk of heart disease (see discussion in chapter 7).

CHAPTER 7

REWRITING THE STARS

For decades, experts believed that our genes were our destiny. You may have been told by your doctor or well-meaning "experts" that your health is largely dependent on your family's history of disease. But in fact, recent studies have shown that our genes have little to do with our life-span or our health span. Instead, the way we live our lives has a greater influence on our well-being over time.

The reality is that much of the aging process, as well as age-related disease, is governed by the state of your mitochondria.[1] And the good news is that the state of your mitochondria is almost entirely within your (and your microbiome's) control. When you use the strategies in this book to stimulate uncoupling, you will see improvements that you may have once thought were out of reach. To borrow a phrase from *The Greatest Showman*, you have the power to rewrite your stars!

You may recall the twin study I shared in chapter 1, in which researchers found that the likelihood to be overweight was based not in genetics, but in mitochondrial health.[2] Consider the implications of this discovery. If you are obese or overweight, as the vast majority of Americans are, this is good news. Your genes are not writing your destiny; your mitochondria are just doing a terrible job of burning the calories in the foods you eat as they convert them into ATP. Instead of literally wasting them via uncoupling, too often the mitochondria are instead sending those calories over to fat storage. No protons are managing to escape the Mito Club's emergency exits. And that's the key difference between the twin who is prone to put on weight easily and the twin who can eat whatever they want and never gain an ounce.

On the Keto Code plan, you will learn how to turn your Prius mitochondria into Ferraris, instructing them to waste fuel with abandon. They will rev up their calorie and fat burning without ATP production to show for it. This will, in turn, stimulate your mitochondria to make more of themselves, as well as prompt them to repair any damage. When you switch on these three processes, losing weight and maintaining great health become effortless. Just like my patient Janet.

Live Long Like a Hummingbird

In the 1920s, Raymond Pearl, an American biologist from Johns Hopkins University, proposed an aging hypothesis called the rate of living theory. Typically, animals that are smaller tend to live shorter lives; for example, fruit flies live for a couple of months—horses, on the other hand, walk the planet for twenty-five to thirty years. Because of this observation, Pearl suggested that every animal had only a specific amount of energy allotted to it, and the faster it was used, the shorter the animal's life would be. It was a popular idea for decades.[3]

There was only one problem with Pearl's theory: birds. Despite their small size—which, by Pearl's logic, should have predicted a very short life-span—birds can live well into old age. Parrots have been known to live into their eighties, while hummingbirds—which only grow to a length of 3 to 4 inches—can live for as long as ten years. At the heart of their long life-spans? Mitochondrial uncoupling. Hummingbirds dip their beaks into flowers to gather their precious nectar, which contains retinoic acid, a type of polyphenol that gives flowers their burst of color. Retinoic acid activates the hummingbirds' uncoupling proteins.[4] Other birds that live longer than their sizes might eat various plants and seeds found on land or in the sea that contain compounds that promote uncoupling.

MITOCHONDRIA AND BRAIN HEALTH

Your brain is an incredibly complex organ. Not only does it govern every thought, feeling, and movement but it is also the only major organ to be composed of about 60 to 70 percent fat. It is primarily made up of two long-chain omega-3 and omega-6 fatty acids, docosahexaenoic acid (DHA) and arachidonic acid (AA), respectively.

The human brain is unique among animals (with the exception of whales and dolphins, but that's another story) in terms of the sheer amounts of DHA and AA it contains. The size of the brain, the size of the hippocampus (the brain's memory center), and even memory function are all correlated to how much DHA is in the bloodstream.

Omega-3 and omega-6 fats are excellent construction material, providing the building blocks for new brain cells. These fats also help neurons function optimally and prompt mitochondrial uncoupling.[5] As you may recall, uncoupling generates heat and produces carbon dioxide (CO_2). Neurons just so happen to appreciate both.[6] The extra heat puts your brain cells into a state that allows them to function more efficiently.[7] And CO_2 has the power to locally dilate blood vessels, which leads to increased blood flow. That's a good thing, because when blood flow in the brain is restricted, it can lead to everything from headaches to (in extreme cases) stroke. In addition, all that extra blood flow facilitates increased energy production. Through mitochondrial uncoupling, all these forces converge to help your brain just plain work better.

Fat Brain Food

Dr. Stephen Cunnane, a preeminent researcher at the University of Sherbrooke in Quebec, has extensively studied the effects of MCT oil on the brain. In 2016, he and his associates published research showing that MCT oil had a positive effect on the brains of Alzheimer's patients. As we will see later in this book, even a mild dose of MCT oil (about 1 tablespoon) has significant positive effects on neuronal activity, even in patients who have brain-related disease. A follow-up study on healthy brains showed a similar benefit, with significant increases in neuron mitochondria activity after supplementation.[8]

Take a Deep Breath

If you've ever hyperventilated, you might have noticed that your fingers and toes went numb. You might've even felt woozy! That's because your neurons weren't getting enough carbon dioxide and couldn't do their jobs well. In fact, when neurosurgeons operate on a patient's brain, it's common practice to induce hyperventilation to lower the amount of CO_2 in their patient's blood. Lower CO_2 translates to slower blood flow and less bleeding—two factors that make for a smoother surgery.

In contrast, individuals who practice breath control, or learning to hold their breath for an extended period, often report heightened perception and cognition. By controlling their breath, they increase the amount of CO_2 in their blood and brain, which increases blood flow to neurons.[9] Despite what you may think, as a heart surgeon, I can assure you that holding your breath for even extended periods of time does not lower your blood oxygen levels, but instead raises CO_2 levels in the blood, which in turn improves neuron function.

Breath control also calms the sympathetic nervous system, which is responsible for the "fight or flight" stress response. When the body is in this meditative state, it further uncouples mitochondria, creating some local heat for neurons and more systemic heat across the body. The body's responses to altered breathing help explain why those trained in breathwork, like Buddhist monks and Wim Hof, demonstrate an enhanced tolerance for freezing temperatures. Hof and monks who regularly practice breathwork have even been known to melt snow and dry wet towels using the heat generated by their bodies, just by changing their breathing patterns.[10] They can thank their uncoupled mitochondria for that extra warmth!

THE KEY(S) TO YOUR HEART

Mitochondrial uncoupling also has distinct benefits for heart health. In a famous study called the Lyon Diet Heart Study, French and

Greek physicians compared the Mediterranean diet with added ALA (a short-chain omega-3 fat found in canola and flaxseed oils) to the American Heart Association's low-fat diet to determine which would be more effective in preventing recurrent heart attacks in individuals who had already suffered a coronary event. They found that the Mediterranean-ALA diet was vastly superior to the low-fat diet—so superior, in fact, that they stopped the trial after three years because it would have been unethical to continue asking study participants to consume the low-fat diet.

Now, I wouldn't blame you for thinking that the Mediterranean-ALA diet's effects were the result of the mainstays of the Mediterranean diet: olive oil and polyphenol-rich plants. I'm certain these nutritious foods did play a vital role in the diet's success. But when the study authors examined the results more closely, they discovered that it was only the amount of ALA circulating in a participant's blood that directly correlated to improved outcomes. The ALA uncoupled mitochondria in the blood vessels, allowing them to nurture and repair the cells' powerhouses.[11] But ALA doesn't just help keep your blood vessels healthy. In another study, an ALA-based high-fat diet prevented weight gain compared to a ketogenic diet high in animal fat.[12] Once again, we can thank mitochondrial uncoupling for such effects. The ALA uncoupled mitochondria, performed a caloric bypass, and wasted calories instead of converting them into ATP. Yet another example that shows why choosing your fats wisely makes such a huge difference when eating a "high fat" diet. When it comes to heart health, a tablespoon of flaxseed oil or canola oil, both rich in ALA, will give you more uncoupling power than, say, a tablespoon of bacon grease.

This effect may be even more pronounced when comparing a high-DHA (that long-chain omega-3 fatty acid mentioned above) diet to the classic keto diet, which is high in omega-6 fats. By enjoying foods with DHA, you get incredible benefits like mitochondrial uncoupling, fat burning, and gene activation for glucose regulation and tumor suppression, just to name a few. When researchers compared omega-3- and omega-6-based diets, they found that the animals that consumed the DHA diet had mitochondria that were over 100 percent more uncoupled, showed 35 percent less fat mass, and had 100 to 340 percent more genes activated for glucose regulation and tumor suppression than the animals who were eating chow high in omega-6s. In addition, the animals showed improvements in their immune function![13] This is great news. When you follow the Keto Code program and choose uncoupling fats over other types of fat, you will see a whole host of fantastic health benefits.

ALA isn't the only uncoupler that benefits heart health—melatonin can help prevent heart disease with uncoupling signals, too. We've known for decades that people who work the night shift have much higher rates of diabetes and heart disease that those who work during the day. Historically, that difference has been attributed to a forced change in circadian rhythm. Recently, researchers at the University of Texas conducted a study to determine whether increasing melatonin production could protect against heart disease. The study authors used genetically engineered mice prone to atherosclerosis—a condition where fats and plaque build up in the arteries of the heart, leading to blockages. When the researchers increased the mice's melatonin levels, either by genetic engineering or supplementation, they were able to prevent their blood vessels from becoming clogged.[14]

Results like these make you reconsider how we discuss melatonin and its role in health. I maintain that we need to stop thinking of it as just a sleep hormone and instead appreciate it as an all-in-one hormone, antioxidant, and uncoupler that helps protect us from disease. You see, this one little hormone is critical to mitochondrial repair work. Certainly, that repair work generally occurs when we are asleep and not eating, but that doesn't mean melatonin's beneficial effects are limited to helping you get some shut-eye. In fact, its effects on our mitochondria are so valuable that regularly adding melatonin-rich foods like pistachios and mushrooms to your diet is, and I use this term intentionally, a no-brainer!

Nicotine: An Unlikely Uncoupler

Let's get one thing straight: smoking cigarettes, or any other tobacco product, is bad for your health and is a known cause of cancer, respiratory disease, and heart disease. As a doctor, I would never in a million years recommend you start smoking cigarettes, and if you do smoke, please stop doing so. Now.

That said, there is an interesting paradox to smoking: some studies have shown that along with its many dangers come some health benefits. One such study of 30,000 British doctors showed that smoking reduced the incidence of Parkinson's disease by a whopping 30 percent.[15] Other research has shown a correlation between smoking and a reduced risk and slowed progression of dementia.[16]

How could it be that something as toxic as cigarette smoke could have protective benefits? The answer lies not in the smoke, but in nicotine, a compound naturally present in tobacco—and a mitochondrial uncoupler.[17] This is perhaps another reason, beyond eating fiber- and polyphenol-rich foods, that Kitavan and European smokers are so thin. And it helps explain why the neurons of smokers are resistant to cognitive decline.

There are ways to ingest nicotine without smoking, of course—from patches to gums to drops—but if you follow the nutritional guidelines of my Keto Code plan, you won't have a need for any such supplements. It's important to remember that even if nicotine is a great uncoupler, it's a greater addiction problem.

UNLOCKING CANCER

Many keto enthusiasts point to the beneficial effects ketones have on the prevention and treatment of cancer.[18] In fact, studies have validated the protective effect of a ketogenic diet against cancer, and in my own clinics, I've seen cancer patients improve dramatically when following the ketogenic version of my Plant Paradox eating plan, which incorporates MCT oil and polyphenol-rich foods and supplements.

How does a keto diet combat cancer? The prevailing theory, first suggested by Dr. Otto Warburg, a twentieth-century German biochemist who won the Nobel Prize for his pioneering work on cellular metabolism, was that ketones "starved" cancer cells of fuel, killing them off. But the more I investigated the mechanisms of keto, the more I became convinced that the uncoupling effect is what rescues dysfunctional mitochondria and helps them protect their cells.[19] Let me explain.

You already know that eukaryotic cells rely on mitochondria to make ATP. As a reminder, eukaryotic cells, or cells with a clearly defined nucleus, evolved more than two billion years ago when ancient primordial cells engulfed bacteria, resulting in a mutually beneficial relationship between the two. In exchange for massive amounts of energy production (the making of ATP), the bacteria got a safe place to stay, with the added bonus of free meals, and eventually developed into mitochondria. Prior to engulfing those bacteria (now mitochondria), ancient primordial cells made their energy currency by glycolysis, the fermentation of protein or sugar, which generates two molecules of ATP from every one molecule of protein or sugar. Compare that to our mitochondria, which can make thirty-two molecules of ATP from the same resources. They don't call them powerhouses for nothing!

If mitochondria are repeatedly damaged by ROSs, or just hammered, over time, by diets high in sugar and fat, energy production will plummet. At that point, the cell will go into a sort of safe operating mode, falling back on those old-school fermenting processes to make ATP instead of trusting the mitochondria to do their job. Over time, existing in this mode will initiate a cascade of processes that override the cell's normal functioning. In fact, fermentation will shut down an important cell function called contact inhibition. In healthy cells, contact inhibition instructs any growing cell to stop dividing and growing when it starts to run into its neighbor. But when the cell is in this safe mode, it will keep growing and dividing no matter how many neighbors are nearby. That's why cancer cells grow so wildly, expanding until they take over entire organs or even run rampant across the entire body.

When you resuscitate damaged mitochondria through uncouplers and get them back "online" in terms of energy production, these abnormal cells no longer need to revert to fermentation to make energy. In theory—and as I've seen in my practice—mitochondrial uncoupling helps fix the problem, allowing the mitochondria to come back online. There's no need for safe mode, or its outdated processes, and the risk of cancer cells spreading is significantly reduced. In fact, cancer cells can revert back into normal cells once mitochondria come back into the fold.

In fact, many "natural" cancer treatment programs promote the use of mitochondrial uncouplers, even if they aren't doing so intentionally and don't refer to them as such. The Budwig diet relies on high-dose flaxseed oil (full of ALA and lignan polyphenols) and a fermented soft cheese called quark. The Gerson therapy uses coffee enemas. The Gonzalez Protocol, brainchild of the recently deceased Dr. Nicholas Gonzalez,[20] and the Hippocrates Health Institute both recommend greens, juicing, and prolonged fasting. When you look at these different therapies, they share two key factors: the use of ketone generation and ingesting uncouplers.

I'd like to offer one more piece of evidence: shift workers don't just have higher rates of diabetes and cardiovascular disease—they also have higher rates of cancer, especially breast cancer. Problems with melatonin production strike again![21] And sure enough, studies show that melatonin has the power to prevent and reverse cancers through uncoupling mechanisms—enhancing mitochondrial function in the process.[22]

To that end, I am now prescribing what many would consider ultra-high doses of melatonin, up to 100mg a day in divided doses, to some of my patients diagnosed with dementia or cancer to help get their mitochondrial function back online. (I'm even using it on our beloved old Labradoodle, Pearl, whom you'll meet in the acknowledgments. We've been giving her 44mg of melatonin a day, along with a host of other uncouplers, for the past year to treat and reverse what our vet had diagnosed as inoperable, obstructive bladder cancer. A year ago, Pearl couldn't empty her bladder. Two weeks after starting her supplements, she started peeing like a racehorse and hasn't had a problem since. I guess you can teach an old dog a new trick.)

The theory of mitochondrial dysfunction as the underlying defect in cancer is a compelling one.[23] It means that, when you follow a diet that promotes uncoupling and the repair of dysfunctional mitochondria, you can help prevent cancer from taking root in the first place.[24] If the chain-smoking Kitavans can live to such ripe old ages and remain cancer and heart disease free, it's certainly worth considering.

Medieval Medicine

I'm an avid student of history. In fact, my special major as an undergrad at Yale was human evolutionary biology, where I examined how changes in food supply and environment shaped the way human beings evolved both physically and socially. Years later, I found myself going down a rabbit hole with regards to the history of the spice trade.

In the Middle Ages, traveling from Europe to Northeast Africa and Asia, or taking a sea route around the tip of Africa to India and the Spice Islands (now part of Indonesia), was an incredibly long and arduous journey. In fact, some historians estimate that 50 percent of traders from Italy, Portugal, Holland, and England during the Middle Ages died in the pursuit of foreign herbs and spices. It begs the question: Why would spice traders take on such a risk?

Certainly, the rarity of spices made them expensive, and the spice trade was a lucrative business. But aside from their culinary value, what made them so coveted? Could it be that their biological effects enhanced their value? Rather than spicing up a meal, was this in fact the first drug trade? Some of the most treasured spices—turmeric, cloves, and ginger—are, notably, rich in polyphenols.

Even before the Middle Ages, many spices had huge value. For example, anyone who has watched a Christmas pageant is familiar with the story of the Three Wise Men, who brought the infant Jesus gold, frankincense, and myrrh. The Bible will tell you these gifts had spiritual meaning. But frankincense and myrrh also have value as mitochondrial uncouplers![25] Both these compounds come from the resin of trees (*Boswellia* and *Commiphora abyssinica*, respectively)— and were used not only to create oils and perfumes, but also different medical ointments with powerful anti-inflammatory and anti-cancer effects. Today we understand their mechanism of action, but the Wise Men knew their value even thousands of years ago.

The same rule applies when you consider the most expensive of all ancient spices: saffron, from the *Crocus sativus* flower—so rare that it was once used as currency (you know the saying "worth its weight in gold"?). Those of you who cook with saffron know that it imparts a very subtle flavor but a rich gold color. But as a mitochondrial uncoupler that fights reactive oxygen species (ROSs) while protecting neurons, it has few equals.[26] In fact, in placebo-controlled trials, saffron was more effective (and better tolerated) than donepezil (Aricept), the most widely prescribed Alzheimer's medication for the treatment of mild to moderate cognitive impairment.[27] That's the kind of spice we could all benefit from!

Take a look at the various polyphenol-rich options—many of which are likely in your spice cabinet right now—in the chart on the following page.

POLYPHENOL-RICH HERBS AND SPICES

This chart ranks herbs and spices from highest to lowest by their respective polyphenol content. Take note: Even thyme, at the bottom of the list, boasts an impressive amount of polyphenols! And certainly any discussion of spices and polyphenols should also include ginger and turmeric. Although these two spices are lower in polyphenols than some of the other spices listed here, both are potent mitochondrial uncouplers as well as mitogenesis promoters.[28] With effects like these, you don't need Simon & Garfunkel to tell you what was being traded down at Scarborough Fair (parsley, sage, rosemary, and thyme—get it?). It was potent polyphenol-rich uncouplers! It would seem the ancients were pretty savvy consumers after all, harnessing the life-enhancing benefits of uncoupling from these remarkable herbs and spices.

Cloves	Rosemary
Cinnamon	Sage
Allspice	Tarragon
Marjoram	Peppercorn
Oregano	Thyme[29]
Mint	

Your health span is not written by your genes; you have the power to eat foods that signal your mitochondria to uncouple and, in doing so, better support your well-being. Before we move on, it's important to note that spices and polyphenols, while direct mitochondrial uncouplers in their own right, are not always well absorbed by the human body. Even so, they remain superb prebiotics for your microbiome, helping them produce critical postbiotics like butyrate as well as other vital SCFAs. Furthermore, the microbiome also helps transform polyphenols in foods and spices into other, more active compounds that can be easily absorbed to signal the mitochondria that it's time to do their uncoupling work.

With that in mind, let's get started on a whole-body tune-up that will jump-start ketone production and optimize your health.

CHAPTER 8

THE NUTRITION PARADOX

Many epidemiological and nutrition studies have shown strong associations between a particular food or diet and the development of a disease (or, in some cases, the prevention of some sort of disease). For example, I have often referred to Ancel Keys's famous Seven Countries Study, which was one of the first to suggest that diet—in particular, saturated fats—plays a role in cardiovascular disease. Keys suggested that a diet high in saturated fats was strongly associated with coronary heart disease deaths, but he could not prove that saturated fats *caused* heart disease.[1]

When Keys began his research, he surveyed the diets of several cultures across the globe, taking note of their different eating patterns and lifestyles—and how such diets might intersect with heart and vascular diseases. Despite the fact that he started off studying the populations of many countries, eventually Keys narrowed his focus to just seven: the United States, Italy, Finland, Yugoslavia, Greece, Japan, and the Netherlands. Based on his research in these regions, he claimed diets high in saturated animal fat significantly increased a person's risk of dying from a heart attack. And when you review his research, it's all too easy to conclude that saturated fat, in fact, *caused* the heart disease. Heck, the US government, as well as most of the medical establishment, immediately embraced this finding and set dietary guidelines accordingly.

But in their rush to protect public health, these officials overlooked an important tenet of scientific research: correlations do not equal causation. Just because people in certain countries eat a lot of saturated fat doesn't mean those diets are directly responsible for cardiovascular disease. There are a host of other factors at play.

Let me explain. When we consider the list of countries Keys chose to study, I can't help but wonder why France didn't make the cut. It's certainly close to Italy and the Netherlands, and France is well-known for its epicurean culture. But the French eat plenty of saturated fat and remain healthy. After all, the French consume twice the amount of cheese and *four times* the amount of butter as Americans do. Yet only 143 out of every 100,000 middle-aged French men die from coronary heart disease.[2] Do you know the statistic for American middle-aged men and coronary heart disease deaths? It's 315 out of 100,000! I suspect the reason France wasn't included in Keys's study is that the data wouldn't have fit his hypothesis. If his argument was correct, French people should have been keeling over from heart attacks left and right.

To complicate matters even further, individuals who hail from Toulouse, a city in the southwest of the country, have the lowest possible risk of dying from coronary heart disease of all the people who reside in France. This is a city that prides itself on goose and duck liver pâtés, duck fat, sausages, and a variety of incredible cheeses. (Having lectured there, I couldn't believe how amazing the local food was!) But despite the prevalence of saturated animal fats, primarily from foods like cheese, butter, and the fatty liver that is the basis of pâté, the risk of heart attack death in Toulouse remains stunningly low.

I mention the Seven Countries Study here not to suggest that it's okay to eat a diet high in saturated fat in order to benefit from ketones. Remember: You can transcend the limitations of the traditional high-fat keto diet, while eating plenty of plant foods, and reap all the mitochondrial benefits of a keto protocol (including weight loss). I'm sharing the Keys study, rather, as an example of what happens when we conflate correlation with causation. So much of what we've been taught about healthy diet stems from associations, not direct causal evidence. And as we move into the Keto Code plan, I want you to consider that some of the rules about healthy eating you may have accepted as nutrition canon aren't as unimpeachable as you may have thought.

For instance, look at all those fats the French are eating. They indulge in dairy products, especially goat's- and sheep's-milk cheeses and butter (butyrate, right?), on a regular basis. Do you see where I'm going here? All these delicious foods are rich sources of MCTs, and in the case of the cheeses, MCTs plus polyamines and the odd-chain fatty acids C15 and 17. It's hard to find a more perfect uncoupling package! So much for dairy fats as a whole being the enemy of health.

Indeed, a new study from late 2021, a continuation of the groundbreaking Framingham Heart Study, the longest dietary and lifestyle trial to date, showed that the consumption of only four fatty acids offered protection from coronary heart disease (and predicted longevity, to boot). Drum roll, please: It probably doesn't surprise you to learn that those good fats included the omega-3 fat docosahexaenoic acid (DHA); palmitoleic acid (C16:1n7), found primarily in macadamia nut oil and sea buckthorn oil; behenic acid (C22), a very-long-chain fatty acid contained in canola oil and, again, macadamia nuts; and, finally, myristic acid (C14), found in coconut and dairy foods. Conclusions? Fats are not the bad guys so many health experts have made them out to be. So take some DHA, munch on those macadamia nuts, and don't shy away from cheese or coconut milk. By eating these foods, you'll uncouple your way to great health![3]

Let's take a look at another correlation/causation mix-up that has governed our thinking about diet. Melatonin is an antioxidant and hormone I heartily recommend to my patients. Yet nearly every time I mention melatonin, they immediately say, "The sleep hormone?" Now, the body's level of melatonin (which is produced by both the pineal gland and our mitochondria) certainly rises as bedtime approaches. And when that happens, you get sleepy. But does that mean melatonin *induces* sleep? It would be an easy correlation/causation mistake to make. But what if our melatonin levels rise to do something else while we slumber? What if an increase in melatonin isn't so much for encouraging sleep, but to induce another critical process that is best accomplished during the sleep cycle? That means sleep and increased melatonin are associated, but doesn't mean sleep causes a spike in melatonin, or vice versa.

You now know that melatonin acts as a "bouncer" at the Mito Club, helping your mitochondria repair themselves. You also know that melatonin can act as an uncoupler of mitochondria in its own right. Maybe that's the hormone's true purpose. After all, you don't eat when you're asleep (hopefully). After a solid 8 hours of not eating, your body will run low on glucose, your insulin levels will fall, and your fat cells will release free fatty acids (FFAs). The FFAs can act as direct mitochondria uncouplers, of course—at least, in cells outside the brain. And certainly, some of those FFAs will head to the liver, where they will be converted into ketones.

But wait, there's more! Now melatonin arrives. The pump has been primed, so to speak—mitochondria are already being nurtured through uncoupling. They are multiplying, sharing their workload, and are ready for the all-important repair work melatonin provides. It all connects over a 24-hour period to help keep your mitochondria in tip-top shape. And in doing so, these different uncouplers come together to promote health and longevity.

Once again, we've made the assumption that correlation is the same as causation—and that's likely why the scientific community missed the importance of mitochondrial uncoupling to weight loss, health, and longevity for so long. Our assumptions had us looking in all the wrong places!

TIME FOR A TUNE-UP

Any beautifully designed entity needs maintenance and upkeep. That includes the human body. Just like a car, you need to follow the manufacturer's guidelines for use and make sure to service your body as required. That's what will keep the warranty valid!

I'm sure your car has some kind of sensor that tells you when your next service is due. Newer cars are now so sophisticated that they can factor in how much wear and tear the vehicle has endured and adjust the service reminder accordingly. You likely have a "check engine" light, too—a warning message that tells you something isn't right. The manufacturer of your car knows exactly how long you can go before maintenance is needed. It also knows when a critical part of the engine is or will soon be failing. (As an aside, I have never been in a NYC taxi that doesn't have the "check engine" light illuminated. Perhaps that says something about the wear and tear on those vehicles!)

Your body, too, has programmed service intervals. I mentioned melatonin earlier for a reason. The service interval for your mitochondria is every 24 hours. While your body rests, uncouplers help to ensure that your mitochondria are getting that much-needed repair work. Furthermore, your body has plenty of built-in "check engine" lights, too. High blood pressure, a high fasting blood glucose level, an elevated HbA1c, erectile dysfunction, depression, autoimmune disease, memory loss, exhaustion, and cancer—just to name a few—are all warnings that maintenance is needed.

And that maintenance starts by taking a long, hard look at your nutrition. Unfortunately, up to 70 percent of the foods Americans eat are highly processed, filled with added sugar, vegetable oils, and preservatives. It's not exactly premium fuel to put in your tank. Too often, we are all too quick to latch onto the current food "enemy" and make the same correlation/causation mistake that Keys made back in the day. Yes, our processed foods are loaded with fats and sugars, but some of the foods that are commonly called out as "bad" may just be innocent bystanders.

For instance, a few of my friends and colleagues are beating their chests over how damaging polyunsaturated fatty acids (PUFAs) are to your health. They now say it's the horrendous amount of linoleic acid (LA), a short-chain omega-6 fat, and alpha-linolenic acid (ALA), a short-chain omega-3 fat, both found in common vegetable oils, that are to blame for rampant inflammation and nearly every serious health condition imaginable.

Not so fast! Both LA and ALA are essential fatty acids. The fact that they are categorized as "essential" means you need them to survive—and since your body doesn't make them on its own, you need to consume them. As it so happens, most of the important lipids in your mitochondria are constructed from these fats. It presents quite a conundrum, doesn't it? Can't live with 'em, can't live without 'em! But as noted in a new paper published by researchers at the prestigious Van Andel Institute in Grand Rapids, Michigan, PUFAs remain important to optimal mitochondrial function, but the ability for mitochondria to use them is thwarted by too much sugar in the diet. More to the point, all that sugar prevents mitochondrial uncoupling. It's easy to say PUFAs are a problem. But here we have a situation where these essential fatty acids are merely guilty by association. It's all that nonessential sugar that's really the issue. The good news is that adopting the Keto Code diet allows mitochondria to make use of these PUFAs again—and supports normal uncoupling processes![4]

You also need to look at *when* and *how* you eat. Most of us are eating 16 hours a day or more. This is a problem, and one that is impacting public health; studies show that 88 percent of middle-aged Americans are insulin resistant. Startlingly, only about one-third of normal-weight adults are metabolically flexible (able to switch from burning glucose to FFAs). In overweight and obese adults, that drops to more like 8 percent and 0.5 percent, respectively.[5] Go ahead, read those lines again and let that information sink in. If you are overweight, 92 percent of you will not be able to shift to fat burning. If you are obese, the percentage rises to 99.5 percent—meaning the vast majority of obese individuals will be unable to make that important switch.

What does this mean? Unfortunately, even when we do stop eating and go to sleep each night, our FFAs, stored in our fat cells, will not be liberated. Our high insulin levels will block that from happening. (Frankly, even if they *were* being released, sky-high insulin levels would prevent your mitochondria from burning them as fuel.) Since the FFAs aren't being released from your fat cells, no ketones are being made, and no signals to uncouple are being sent to your mitochondria. No caloric bypass. No mitogenesis. No repair.

Worse yet, consistently high insulin levels will prevent glucose from getting where it's needed in the body. As a result, your brain goes hungry at night when ketones should be fueling your neurons until morning. In addition, without ketones to signal that all-important uncoupling "repair mode," your neurons are left in disrepair (no uncoupling means no cleanup at the Mito Club!). Over time, your neurons become increasingly damaged and may die, leading to cognitive decline. You should consider any cognitive impairment or neurological symptoms a bright red flashing "check engine" light!

DOUBLE-CHECK YOUR INSURANCE POLICY

If you're going to invest in a full body tune-up, you probably want to make sure you're not putting your vehicle at risk unnecessarily—and many of us make choices every day that undermine our best efforts at keeping our parts in working order. In addition to consuming too much, too often, it's also important to be aware of seemingly small factors that impact mitochondrial health. For example, common blood pressure medications like beta-blockers can suppress melatonin production by up to 80 percent.[6] Other widely used drugs, such as broad-spectrum antibiotics, nonsteroidal anti-inflammatory drugs (NSAIDs), and stomach-acid blockers, also prevent uncoupling. But even if you don't take a single prescription or over-the-counter drug, there are two environmental influences that harm mitochondrial function and are absolutely essential to avoid: blue light and the herbicide glyphosate (also known by the brand name Roundup).

The Unseen Damage of NSAIDs

If you're familiar with any of my Paradox books, you may recall that one of the Seven Deadly Disruptors, or factors that cause a leaky gut and excess inflammation, is the overuse of NSAIDs like aspirin, ibuprofen (Advil), and naproxen (Aleve). In one book, I actually likened them to hand grenades with the power to blow holes in your gut wall! (I stand by that statement.)

How do they wreak such havoc in the gut? When absorbed into the intestinal wall, NSAIDs dramatically uncouple the mitochondria of the cells lining that wall. They do so with the same force and power of DNP, that dangerous weight-loss drug—they've even been compared to DNP in certain studies.[7] That kind of overwhelming uncoupling response caused those cells to die due to a severe lack of ATP, which in turn leaves a gaping hole in the gut wall. This is yet another example, and a rather dramatic one, that in uncoupling, a little dab will do ya. If you aren't careful, you can have too much of a good thing.

The blue light emitted from our cell phones, LED lights, computers, and TV screens directly increases ROS generation in our retinas and prevents appropriate protective mitochondrial uncoupling. Over time, this causes macular degeneration. Glyphosate (Roundup), a toxin sprayed on conventional crops as a desiccant herbicide prior to harvest, not only harms our microbiome and causes leaky gut, but—no surprise—disrupts uncoupling mechanisms directly, including the mitochondria's ability to repair themselves.[8] Such disruptors should be avoided at all costs, and though they are omnipresent in our lives, it *is* possible to avoid them. Get yourself a pair of blue-blocking glasses for looking at screens at night, and eliminate all blue light from your bedroom when you sleep. To avoid ingesting glyphosate, try to choose organic foods and wines as much as possible.

Here's the good news: even the most broken-down machines can usually be repaired, or at least be made to run a bit smoother. Because so much damage has occurred, you will need more than a simple oil change (the equivalent of going on a cleanse or a two-week weight loss program) to get your mitochondria back into tip-top shape. You need a full tune-up. That's exactly what we are going to do shortly.

The Keto Code plan will harness the power of MCTs to create uncoupling ketones even when insulin levels are high. The plan will give your microbiome the fiber it needs to produce uncoupling postbiotics like butyrate. It will slowly shorten your eating window to enhance ketone and FFA production. And by consuming polyphenol-rich foods and spices, you will turn your broken-down Prius into a mint-condition Ferrari—uncoupling not only to survive, but to thrive.

Let the tune-up begin!

CHAPTER 9

THE KETO CODE PROGRAM

The objective of the Keto Code program is to find your sweet spot—that Goldilocks place where just enough mitochondria uncouple to support your health and weight loss goals, without going overboard. When you eat foods that feed your microbiome (and, consequently, uncouple and stimulate your mitochondria), you can heal your gut, reduce inflammation, and rev up your mitochondria's ability to waste fuel and thus help you lose weight. The key factor here is that you're choosing foods to both promote ketone production and support mitochondrial function. That means you'll be able to enjoy a much wider array of foods than you would on a traditional ketogenic diet.

Not only will we make some changes to *what* you eat, we're also going to make adjustments to *when* you eat. By following my time-restricted eating protocol—which I refer to as chrono-consumption—you will give your mitochondria the overhaul they need to improve metabolic flexibility, boost insulin sensitivity, increase your energy levels, and improve your overall health.

The eating program itself is pretty straightforward—we'll get there in a minute. But before we do, let's take a closer look at the three goals of this program:

1. **Create ketones:** Practicing time-restricted eating will help to release free fatty acids (FFAs) from fat cells, which will in turn generate ketones in the liver. And consuming MCT oil or MCT-containing foods like goat's- or sheep's-milk products will generate ketones directly.

2. **Rejuvenate the microbiome:** You will feed your gut buddies plenty of prebiotics in the form of soluble fiber, which will enable the production of postbiotics. Furthermore, vinegars and other fermented products provide a direct shot of postbiotics (yes, postbiotics, not probiotics) that have been shown to dramatically rehabilitate your likely decimated microbiome.[1] But if you need to supplement, you can also buy preformed postbiotics directly (my recommended supplements are listed in the appendix on page 225).

3. **Uncouple with plant polyphenols:** Consuming foods rich in polyphenols and other plant-based nutrients will boost mitochondrial uncoupling.

When you eat in accordance with those guidelines, a wide array of foods is available to you. I'm not going to make you eat anything you don't want to eat; this program was created with flexibility and options in mind. Whether you are vegetarian or an omnivore, a Paleo devotee or a hardcore vegan, you can eat well and actually *enjoy* food again. I'm simply asking you to expand your horizons so you can eat for the health of your microbiome and your mitochondria—which, of course, ultimately means *your* health.

When you give your gut buddies the foods they like—greens, jicama, artichokes, or ground flaxseeds, just to name a few examples—your good gut bacteria will return the favor by multiplying, crowding out the bad guys, and restoring balance to your microbiome. (Eliminating artificial sugars and bad fats, which, sadly, make up a predom-

inant part of the traditional keto diet, is also part of this equation.)
That's why this eating plan is focused on the three Ps: probiotics,
prebiotics, and postbiotics. By feeding prebiotics (fermentable fibers
and polyphenols from plants) to probiotics (your gut buddies), they
will produce postbiotics (the SCFAs and gases that act as signaling
compounds) that have the power to heal your gut wall, protect your
brain, and, of course, uncouple your mitochondria for weight loss,
increased energy levels, and improved short- and long-term health!

This new regimen will also harness the power of ketones and
FFAs. These vital signaling molecules get your mitochondria's attention, instructing them to actively uncouple. Here's where this
program really differs from traditional keto diets: you want just the
right amount of ketones and FFAs to get the best results. Most of us
don't make any ketones within a 24-hour period. That's bad enough.
But—keto spoiler alert!—being in a constant state of ketosis is even
worse. It can make your body even *more* inflamed and insulin resistant.[2] That's why keto-consumption is an essential element of this
program. It will allow your body to hit that sweet spot where it makes
enough ketones to promote metabolic flexibility instead of preventing it.

WHAT'S ON THE MENU?

You may be thinking, "Sounds good, Dr. Gundry. But what does this
actually look like on my dinner plate?" Obviously, the more whole
foods you can eat, well, whole, the better. You want to fill your plate
with lots of vegetables that contain both prebiotic fiber and polyphenols. You can also enjoy nuts and some seeds; sheep's- and goat's-
milk dairy products; pressure-cooked lentils and other legumes; some
wild fish, shellfish, and mollusks; and, if you desire, pastured poultry,
omega-3 eggs, and some grass-fed, grass-finished beef, lamb, pork,

or game. It also means some *occasional* prebiotic, in-season, low-fructose fruit—or adopting the practice of reverse juicing (see page 123) all year round.

You can also thrive on this eating plan without consuming animal-sourced foods. In fact, I encourage you to limit your animal protein! But the choice is yours. Heck, I'll even throw in a glass of red wine or champagne at dinner and a piece of extra-dark chocolate or my delicious uncoupling ice cream (see page 213) for dessert. On this plan, the foods you eat may be a bit different from those you usually consume, whether you are currently eating keto or following some other diet, but I promise you, everything will be delicious.

DOS AND DON'TS OF THE KETO CODE PROGRAM

The Keto Code program builds on my previous Paradox eating regimens. As in those, you'll aim to avoid gut-busting lectins at all costs, but you'll also add foods to your diet that stimulate the production of ketones even when you're not fasting. As you scan the food lists at the end of this chapter, you'll notice that may of the "Yes, Please" foods from my previous books are, in fact, uncouplers. To guide your choices and help you incorporate these foods into your meals, I've created a list of dos and don'ts.

Do: Eat Prebiotic Fiber-Rich Plant Foods

Many of you may already be taking a probiotic supplement to support microbiome health. But while supplementation is helpful, feeding your gut buddies the prebiotic fibers they crave is even better. When you eat these foods, you can better reach the good bugs that have been cowering in the far reaches of your gut, sidelined because they lack the nutrients they need to do their jobs. Eating foods that are rich in soluble (and some insoluble) fibers, including tubers, rutabagas, parsnips, radishes, root vegetables, radicchio, endive, okra, artichokes, pressure-cooked beans and legumes, basil seeds, flaxseed, psyllium, and more, supports the health and reproduction of healthy bacteria in your gastrointestinal tract. When your gut buddies get the sustenance they want, they'll tell your brain their needs are being met. As a result, you will literally feel less hungry and begin to crave healthier foods.

By consuming foods rich in prebiotic fiber, you'll make those good bacteria happy, and they'll return the favor by not only nourishing you but uncoupling your mitochondria. In fact, recent studies have found that when individuals who were on a water fast were given about 100 calories of indigestible (for us, at least) prebiotic fiber daily as their only food, they were able to easily continue their fast for seven to fourteen days without experiencing hunger.[3] Consider that for a moment. Here's a situation where the gut buddies got the sustenance they needed. Even though the study participants couldn't digest it, those bugs dined on that fiber, produced postbiotics, and sent the right messages to assure their host that everything was fine. No need to look for any more food!

One of the best prebiotics is inulin, a type of dietary fiber found in foods like chicory, asparagus, onions, leeks, and artichokes. One of my preferred sweeteners, Just Like Sugar (a great sugar substitute for baking) is essentially pure inulin. Both Just Like Sugar and a newer sweetener called allulose offer that sweeter taste without spiking your blood sugar—and they do so while also feeding your gut buddies with prebiotics. Win-win.

Another great way to consume prebiotics is to take psyllium husk powder or, my new favorite, soaked basil seeds. As many of you know, chia seeds are loaded with lectins. But basil seeds give all the benefits of forming a prebiotic gel without the dangers of chia lectins.

Start with a teaspoon a day, mixed in water or not, and work up to a daily tablespoon, or even two, for maximum effect.

Don't: Eat Lectin-Rich Plant Foods

While it's important to eat plant foods rich in prebiotic fiber, it's equally important to avoid lectin-heavy veggies, grains, and improperly prepared legumes. When high-lectin foods were first introduced to the human diet about ten thousand years ago, our health dramatically changed for the worse. Although many people still wouldn't know a lectin from a lemon, my work and that of others has shown they are a danger to our health. Here are just a few reasons why:

1. **Lectins damage digestive and immune health.** Lectins are a plant's defense against being eaten. As such, your gastrointestinal tract has trouble breaking them down. This impairs digestion, reduces nutrient absorption, inflames your immune system, and disrupts the balance in your microbiome.

2. **Lectins create a leaky gut.** Lectins produce holes in your intestinal walls and leak into your bloodstream; the result of these breaches is chronic body-wide inflammation. Once your gut wall has been made permeable, lectins can go on to damage your internal organs and joint tissues. And as my research, as well as that of Dr. Alessio Fasano at Harvard, has shown, the damage from lectins can lead to autoimmune disorders including rheumatoid arthritis, Hashimoto's thyroiditis, diabetes, and coronary artery disease.[4]

3. **Lectins lead to weight gain.** Lectins like wheat germ agglutinin (WGA, a lectin found in whole wheat) stick to insulin receptors on fat cells. In doing so, they prevent leptin, the hormone that controls your appetite, from telling your brain "I'm full!" The

result? You just keep eating. This blockage also signals your body to keep storing fat. When you put the two together, you have a perfect recipe for weight gain.

So what are some common sources of plant-based lectins? There are many—among them are nightshade vegetables (white potatoes, tomatoes, peppers, eggplant, goji berries), brown rice, beans and lentils, grains, and pseudograins (like amaranth, quinoa, and buckwheat), peanuts, cashews, and chia seeds. The good news is that most lectin-containing foods can be consumed after being pressure cooked. (You always knew that Instant Pot was a worthwhile investment!)

The Many Benefits of a Healthy Gut

The inner lining of your gut is covered in a thick layer of mucus. I know that might sound gross, but that mucus helps protect your gut from invaders like lectins. The thicker the mucus, the better!

A family of bacteria called *Akkermansia muciniphila* live in your gut. Not only do these guys reside in the mucus layer, they dine on it (*muciniphila* literally means "mucus loving"). When they chow down, they signal your intestinal mucosal cells, known as enterocytes, to kick up production and make *more* mucus. The more *muciniphila* in your gut lining, the less likely you are to suffer from obesity, inflammation, or diabetes.

In dietary studies, researchers have noticed an interesting side effect. The more a person's eating window is time-restricted, the longer ketones are present, or the higher consumption of polyphenols, the more *muciniphila* appear in the gut. Not only does this result in the production of more mucus, but the presence of these bacteria is also associated with thermogenesis and the conversion of white fat to beige fat. And wouldn't you know it, they also help uncouple mitochondria in gut-lining cells.[5] That's likely why in fruit flies, the presence of *muciniphila* directly correlates with improved longevity.[6] In exciting news, Akkermansia capsules are now becoming available, after considerable research and effort.

Do: Eat Whole Foods

There are all manner of delicious, lectin-free options on the menu—but most of these foods are best consumed whole. Whole foods provide the gut with more resistant starches, which not only better satisfy *your* hunger but that of your gut buddies as well.

A starch is considered "resistant" when it is slowly digested. Because these types of foods "resist" quick digestion, they can make it past your small intestine without significant digestion and absorption there and get into your large intestine, where your gut buddies can convert them into postbiotics like butyrate. Yams, taro root, sorghum, millet, pressure-cooked rice, and cassava can all be transformed into resistant starches when they are cooked, chilled, and reheated.

The more plant material remains in its original form—whole, if you will—the more resistant it will be to digestion (and, as such, more usable for your gut buddies). A yam that was cooked, cooled, and reheated is going to be much more resistant than sweet potato flour or pasta. So, while a cassava flour tortilla is vastly preferable to a traditional wheat flour or corn tortilla (which have high lectin content), it still delivers a whopping load of quickly digested sugars, which won't help with ketone generation. It's always better to eat foods in their unprocessed state.

I should also add that popular root vegetables, like beets and carrots, contain multiple complex carbohydrates and resistant starches—when they are raw. Unfortunately, if you cook them, even a little bit, they lose those components.

Don't: Eat Frankenfoods Loaded with Frankenfats

The most important rule when it comes to your diet is to choose whole foods over processed ones. Unfortunately, the typical American diet is filled with highly processed foods—and all the chemicals, sugars, and fats that come with them. We have known for some time that such a diet is not only pro-inflammatory but also takes a toll on mitochondrial health.[7] Fast foods are typically full of polyunsaturated omega-6 fats from soybean and corn oils, which destroys your ability to make hydrogen sulfide, a postbiotic gasotransmitter that helps alleviate inflammation in the gut.[8]

Processed and fried foods are also hidden sources of trans fats, those now banned fats that somehow still sneak into our food supply. This type of fat, created through industrial processing, clogs the inner membranes of your mitochondria, not only stifling energy production, but making uncoupling nearly impossible. Studies have shown a direct link between trans fats and poor cardiovascular health, unlike the correlations between saturated fats and cardiac events. Is it any wonder they've been linked to higher incidences of heart attack and stroke?

Finally, processed foods are chock-full of chemicals like food colorings, artificial sweeteners, and high-fructose corn syrup. These additives may help these foods look more appealing (and keep them shelf-stable longer), but they take a toll on our health. I have a huge glass jar of Oreos on our countertop at home that has sat there, untouched, for five years. They are as pristine-looking as the day they were made. Not only will I not touch them, but neither will any insects, molds, or bacteria. Nothing will come near them. It's a scary Frankenfood indeed!

Long story short: You want to avoid the additives and preservatives in processed foods at all costs. As just one example of many, titanium dioxide, a common additive used as a whitening agent in personal care products like sunscreens, as well as in the powdered sugary topping found on many doughnuts, has been shown to alter the composition of your microbiome and cause inflammation, especially in your colon.[9]

Do: Get Your Sweetness Naturally

I'm sure many of you have a sweet tooth—in fact, many of the questions I receive about my nutrition programs involve how to satiate those cravings in a healthy way. I recommend only eating fruit in season—and in moderation.

There's a reason fruit is often served for dessert: it's as sweet as candy! In fact, fruit is full of fructose, one of the biggest troublemakers for your mitochondria and liver. And now, thanks to hybridization, fruit is bred to boost its sugar content. When you see apples like the Honeycrisp or Ambrosia, the names give it away—they're pure sugar. In fact, a single apple has a fructose content equivalent to 6 teaspoons of table sugar. That fructose, like table sugar, makes a beeline for your liver, slashing ATP production.[10]

What about berries, you might ask? These days, people talk about berries, especially blueberries, as superfoods. But believe it or not, the modern blueberry actually has the highest sugar content of any berry. Like apples, they're now being bred for more sweetness. So if you're going to eat berries, go for wild blueberries, usually found in the frozen food section. From there, select blackberries, followed by raspberries, then strawberries.

That said, there are some fruits that offer great health benefits with fewer drawbacks. When in season, pomegranate and passion fruit seeds have a very low sugar content and powerful uncoupling benefits. Kiwifruit (skin-on, please! It's loaded with fiber and polyphenols) and grapefruit are both low in sugar and laden with uncoupling polyphenols. In fact, the white pith of a grapefruit—or any other citrus fruit—is loaded with quercetin, an uncoupler. Other polyphenols in citrus and citrus peel have neuroprotective qualities because of their uncoupling effects on neurons.[11]

I suggest treating fruit like dessert—and aim to only eat local and organic varieties, when they're in season (in season depends on where you live, but remember: strawberries have been genetically bred to produce in January here in California, though they are clearly not "legal" then). When it comes to fruit juice, please skip it altogether. Drinking juice is basically mainlining fructose. You always want to opt for the whole fruit.

Reverse Juicing

Giving up fruit can be a real challenge. If you're a fruit lover, one way to get more of the benefits and fewer of the drawbacks is to try a technique I refer to as reverse juicing.

Get out your juicer—I know there's one hiding somewhere in your kitchen—or buy an inexpensive one. Throw in some thawed frozen organic berries, juice them . . . and then throw out the juice!

You heard me right. Toss it right down the sink! I'm basically asking you to do a caloric bypass on your fruit.

Once you've rid yourself of the juice (which, for the record, contains most of the fructose), enjoy the leftover pulp. You can eat it on its own or stir it into your goat's-, sheep's-, or coconut milk yogurt. It's a great dessert, of course, but it's also a wonderful treat to have for your first meal of the day. You'll generate ketones from the MCTs in the yogurt and enjoy concentrated polyphenols to boot. It's a double hit of mitochondrial uncouplers! Get a silicone ice cube tray and freeze the pulp to make an ice cream–like treat for dessert by blending the cubes with the yogurt!

Don't: Eat Sugar

The majority of processed foods contain highly refined sugars and carbohydrates. To understand how much sugar is really contained in popular foods, you must look beyond the grams of sugar listed on the nutrition label. For instance, you can find labeling on some bagels that claims they contain zero grams of sugar. But the industrial milling process transforms wheat into a rapidly available sugar—in fact, an amount equivalent to 8 to 9 teaspoons of table sugar. White bread has a glycemic index rating of 100, which is actually higher than that of table sugar. How can that be? It's because those individual starch molecules are instantly absorbable as sugar.

"But wait," you might say, "there's no listing of *that* sugar on the label." You are 100 percent correct. The label guidelines are designed to hide that kind of sugar content from the consumer. As such, reading labels won't tell you what will happen in your body when you consume these foods. In order to get the real sugar value, you need to subtract the number of grams of fiber (the good stuff for your gut buddies) from the total grams of carbs listed on the label. Then, for fun, further divide that number by 4 to get the equivalent teaspoons of table sugar per serving. (This math will provide you with the sugar content in a single serving . . . but don't forget to look at the serving size listed on the food label—it's probably much smaller than you think. This is another trick food manufacturers have devised to hide the amount of sugar in their products.)

It's important to remember that high-fructose corn syrup is still present in many prepackaged foods, including energy bars, granola bars, and cookies. When you see the words *corn syrup, brown rice syrup, all-natural syrup, cane syrup, or maple syrup* on the ingredient list, you should know they are all code words for fructose, a primary mitochondrial killer you should try to avoid at all costs.

Luckily for those of us with a sweet tooth, there are healthy ways to satisfy it. See page 153 for a list of my favorite sugar substitutes. (Note: These are natural sweeteners, not chemical sweeteners like sucralose, aspartame, and saccharine, which kill gut bacteria and cause inflammation.)[12] Just remember the Goldilocks rule with any sweetener: When you use too much, your brain is tricked into thinking real sugar is coming. When that sugar doesn't appear, your brain will signal you to hunt down something sweet and keep eating. If you find it difficult to go cold turkey on sugar, I suggest weaning yourself off it over a few weeks.

Do: Enjoy Healthy Fats

Your mitochondria need two special substances to protect them from oxidative stress—our Mito Club bouncer melatonin, as well as a range of healthy fats, including phospholipids, a special type of fat molecule found in egg yolks, fish, and other foods. We've already talked about why it's so important to include melatonin in your diet.

While your gut buddies can make this substance from amino acids, a boost of food-sourced melatonin ensures there's extra security detail at the Mito Club. Luckily, eating your melatonin couldn't be easier or more delicious. The foods on the list below contain high levels of melatonin. Please pressure cook, cool, and reheat the rices below.

MELATONIN-RICH FOODS

Melatonin not only acts as a "bouncer," helping your mitochondria deal with excess ROSs; it also works as an uncoupler in its own right. The following foods contain high levels of melatonin (listed from highest to lowest melatonin content).[13]

Pistachios	Red wine
Mushrooms	Cranberries
Black pepper	Almonds
Red rice	Basmati rice
Black rice	Purslane
Mustard seeds	Tart cherries
Olive oil	Strawberries
Brewed coffee	Flaxseed

Now let's get to those healthy fats. Phospholipids and the short- and long-chain omega-3 and long-chain omega-6 fatty acids help keep mitochondrial membranes in tip-top shape to ensure that ATP production can function without a hitch. In addition, these fats house the uncoupling proteins in the mitochondrial membranes, even as they promote uncoupling themselves.

Luckily, these fats are plentiful in shellfish like mussels, scallops, clams, oysters, shrimp, crab, squid, and lobster. Omega-3 egg yolks also have generous amounts of omega-3s, as well as being a rich source of arachidonic acid (AA), a type of omega-6 fatty acid.[14] Olive oil is also a great source of the fats and polyphenols you need to keep your mitochondria—and your overall health—in tip-top shape. In fact, one landmark study found that consuming a liter of olive oil each week helps protect individuals from cardiovascular problems, as well as dementia.[15]

Don't: Overdo It on the Protein

There's a reason so many weight loss programs are centered on protein: it requires a lot of calories to digest. In fact, we lose about 30 percent of the calories in protein just to digestion and heat generation. Given that most of us eat on calorie overload, any opportunity to burn a lot of protein calories while generating heat is beneficial when it comes to weight loss. High-protein diets like the original Atkins plan work by thermogenesis, burning tons of calories in the process of breaking down that protein into its component amino acids.

Given the success many people have had with high-protein diets, you may wonder why you shouldn't follow suit. The problem is that over the long term, high-protein diets deprive your gut buddies of the essential fiber they need to produce SCFAs—those molecules that are so critical for mitochondrial health. In fact, mitochondrial function generally starts to plummet within days of starting a high-protein diet.[16] The production of SCFAs significantly drops,[17] suppressing butyrate production while increasing production of damaging compounds.[18]

Furthermore, overconsumption of animal protein can cause *too* much hydrogen sulfide to be produced in the colon, which ultimately damages your colon cells.[19] Once again, we see the Goldilocks Rule in effect: there can be too much of a good thing. And, of course, when you eat a diet high in animal protein—as is common in most traditional ketogenic diets—you deprive your body of polyphenols, those ultimate uncouplers.

If you enjoy animal protein, I recommend including wild fish and shellfish in your diet. The smaller the fish, the better. Sardines, herring, and anchovies, as well as wild salmon and bivalves (clams, oysters, mussels, and the like) are all great sources of omega-3 fatty acids and phospholipids without the risk of mercury or other heavy metals. Just be sure to avoid "organic" farm-raised salmon, which are fed corn and soybean meal. Thanks to their diet, farmed salmon no longer make DHA, instead producing inflammatory omega-6 fatty acids.

Omega-3 eggs are another good option for most people, but, admittedly, a number of my autoimmune patients do react to the proteins in both the whites and the yolks. When it comes to meat, please enjoy smaller amounts (a maximum of 4 ounces) of the highest-quality meat you can get—and by that I mean 100% grass-fed and grass-finished beef or pasture-raised chicken. These meats will be free of microbiome-disrupting antibiotics, hormones, pesticides, and biocides. (Take note: There's a big difference between "grass-fed" and "grass-fed and grass-finished." There is no federal definition of "grass-fed," so any animal that's eaten some grass on any day of its life can be given the label.)

As for dairy products, my devoted Paradox readers already know the score. Most cow's-milk products in the United States come from a breed of cow that produces milk with a highly inflammatory protein called A1 beta-casein. That's why I recommend you choose goat's- or sheep's-milk dairy products, or cow's-milk dairy from southern European (A2 beta-casein) cows.

Remember, goat, sheep, and water buffalo cheeses and yogurts come with the extra benefit of ketone-generating medium-chain triglycerides (MCTs). They also contain compounds called milk-fat globule membranes (MFGMs). MFGMs surround the fats in these milks and make them soluble. Exciting new research in humans shows that ingesting MFGMs leads to weight loss and reduced insulin resistance.[20] Why? As if you even need to ask at this point! MFGMs are mitochondrial uncouplers.[21]

One note of caution for readers who have been diagnosed with an autoimmune disorder: While more than 90 percent of people with autoimmune disease go into remission on my Plant Paradox program, the 10 percent who don't do well on it usually test positive for reacting to *all* forms of dairy, including A2 beta-casein, and both egg whites and egg yolks.[22]

Please note that there's no need to default to meat as a "must have" protein source. You can find more than ample protein in a plant-rich plate of food. For example, there are 2 grams of protein in almost every serving of vegetables that you can name. I encourage you to consider healthy low-lectin plant protein, whether it be pressure-cooked lentils (with a whopping 18 grams of protein and 15 grams of dietary fiber per cup) or hemp tofu, which contains all the essential amino acids. Textured vegetable protein (TVP), which is pressure- and high-heat-extruded, defatted soy, and hydrolyzed pea and bean proteins and protein isolates of peas and beans are safe to consume,[23] but please read the label carefully before diving in. Pea, bean, and soy proteins that haven't been treated in this way are still chock-full of lectins. Many people can also enjoy plant-based protein sources like spirulina algae protein, flaxseed protein, and hemp protein powders. Nuts are another good source of plant-based protein, with anywhere from 4 to 9 grams of protein, plus all the essential amino acids, per 1-ounce serving.

Do: Eat Postbiotic-Producing Foods

When you eat foods that promote postbiotic production, you're giving your cells the compounds they need to send uncoupling signals. Cruciferous vegetables like broccoli, cauliflower, and other sulfur-containing veggies including onions, garlic, leeks, chives, shallots, and scallions (all part of the allium family) get top billing in this quest to create more of these all-important signaling molecules. Cruciferous veggies also contain compounds that your gut bacteria can convert into indole, a specific type of postbiotic that, among other things, can help prevent fatty liver disease via mitochondrial uncoupling.[24]

Here's a tip when it comes to cruciferous veggies: always chop them before cooking to release myrosinase, an enzyme with important anticancer properties. It gets its cancer-fighting power by producing sulforaphane, which is itself a powerful mitochondrial uncoupler.[25] This enzyme isn't released if you cook the veggies before chopping them.

POLYPHENOL-RICH FOODS

You don't have to look too hard to find foods that are chock-full of polyphenols. Whether you prefer coffee to tea, grapes to berries, or spinach to kale, the plant kingdom is full of delicious polyphenol-rich options to suit any palate, though it's important to also consider the sugar and grain levels of these foods before consuming. While polyphenols can help boost mitochondrial uncoupling, not all of these fit with a Keto Code diet. With that in mind, here's a list of common foods sorted by their polyphenol content, ranked from highest to lowest.[26]

Cloves	Rosemary, dried
Peppermint, dried	Spearmint, dried
Star anise	Common thyme, dried
Cocoa powder	Lowbush blueberry
Mexican oregano	Blackcurrant
Celery seed	Capers
Black chokeberry	Black olive
Dark chocolate	Highbush blueberry
Flaxseed meal	Hazelnut
Black elderberry	Pecan nut
Chestnut	Soy flour
Common sage, dried	Plum

Green olive	Common thyme, fresh
Sweet basil, dried	Refined maize flour
Curry powder	Tempeh
Sweet cherry	Whole-grain rye flour
Globe artichoke	Apple
Blackberry	Spinach
Roasted soybean	Shallot
Milk chocolate	Lemon verbena, dried
Strawberry	Black tea
Red chicory	Red wine
Red raspberry	Green tea
Coffee, filter	Soy yogurt
Ginger, dried	Yellow onion
Whole grain hard wheat flour	Soy meat
	Whole-grain wheat flour
Prune	Apple juice (100% juice)
Almond	Pomegranate juice (100% juice)
Black grape	
Red onion	Extra-virgin olive oil
Green chicory	Black bean

Peach

Blood orange juice
 (100% juice)

Cumin

Grapefruit juice (100% juice)

White bean

Chinese cinnamon

Blond orange juice
 (100% juice)

Broccoli

Red currant

Tofu

Pure lemon juice

Whole grain oat flour

Apricot

Caraway

Refined rye flour

Asparagus

Walnut

Potato

Ceylon cinnamon

Parsley, dried

Nectarine

Curly endive

Marjoram, dried

Red lettuce

Chocolate beverage
 with milk

Quince

Endive (escarole)

Soy milk

Pumelo juice (100% juice)

Rapeseed oil

Pear

Soybean sprout

Green grape

Carrot

Vinegar

Soy cheese

White wine

Rosé wine

What's so striking about this list of foods is not only that we see so many of the spices we just discussed high up on it, but it also contains quite a few new-world foods like cacao, dark chocolate, and Mexican oregano. Truly, there are so many ways to add polyphenol-rich mitochondrial uncouplers to your diet so that you can continue to enjoy the flavors you love.

Take note of how highly ranked flaxseeds and olives are—both foods are easily added to your plate on the Keto Code program. And while not on this list, yerba mate, yet another popular new-world beverage, has also been shown to uncouple mitochondria and signal them to start multiplying.[27] Drink up!

Don't: Eat Foods That Harm Your Gut Buddies

In our never-ending quest to find fast and convenient foods, we do our health a disservice. First and foremost, we need to eat food that feeds our microbiome rather than destroys it. Since they are raised in overcrowded conditions, factory-farmed meats and seafoods (this includes farmed salmon and most shrimp) are fed antibiotics to prevent diseases. Those drugs also help the animals grow faster and faster. Unfortunately, those antibiotics are then incorporated into the animal's flesh, which we eat—and they decimate our gut buddies in the process.

Similarly, a single packet of an artificial sweetener like sucralose (Splenda) has the power to kill half the intestinal bacteria living in your gut. As I've noted in my previous books, artificial sweeteners do far more harm than good. These sweeteners are commonly found in many low-calorie and keto products on the market, including popular keto bars and drinks. This is why it's so important to read the label before taking that first bite or sip.

Finally, your gut is also home to some potentially harmful bacteria. When our gut buddies are well nourished, we don't have to worry about them. But unfortunately, the bad guys thrive on saturated fats and simple sugars. When you make these types of foods mainstays of your diet, you give sustenance to the bad bacteria, allowing them to grow and produce inflammatory lipopolysaccharides (LPSs, or, as I often refer to them, little pieces of shit). The end result is that the bad bacteria grow in size and number, starving out all those good bacteria you rely on and destroying your mitochondria in the process.

THE KETO CODE FOOD LISTS

Okay, dear reader, here are the lists you've been waiting for. The following "yes" and "no" lists comprise the backbone of the Keto Code program. Consider these lists of specific foods and brands as complementing the dos and don'ts you read earlier, and as great quick-and-easy reference tools. As always, you can find this information online at DrGundry.com, where you can download the lists in PDF form.

Yes, Please: Postbiotic-Boosting Foods

Cruciferous Vegetables

Arugula

Bok choy

Broccoli

Brussels sprouts

Cabbage, green and red

Cauliflower

Collards

Kale

Kimchi

Kohlrabi

Napa cabbage

Sauerkraut (raw)

Swiss chard

Watercress[28]

Other Postbiotic-Boosting Vegetables

Artichokes

Asparagus

Bamboo shoots

Beets (raw)

Carrot greens

Carrots (raw)

Celery

Chicory

Chives

Daikon radish

Endive

Escarole

Fiddlehead ferns

Frisée

Garlic

Garlic scapes

Ginger[29]

Hearts of palm

Horseradish

Jerusalem artichokes (sunchokes)

Leeks

Lemongrass

Mushrooms

Nopales (cactus paddles; if you can't find locally, buy online)

Okra

Onions

Parsnips

Puntarelle

Radicchio

Radishes

Rutabaga

Scallions

Shallots

Water chestnuts

Leafy Greens

Basil

Butter lettuce

Cilantro

Dandelion greens

Endive

Escarole

Fennel

Frisée

Mesclun (baby greens)

Mint

Mizuna

Mustard greens

Parsley

Perilla

Purslane

Red- and green-leaf lettuces

Romaine lettuce

Sea vegetables

Seaweed and algae

Spinach

Fruits That Act Like Fats

Avocado (up to a whole one per day)

Olives, all types

Uncoupling Oils

Avocado oil (some effect)

Black seed oil

Canola oil (non-GMO, organic only!)

Coconut oil (some effect)

Cod liver oil (the lemon and orange flavors have no fish taste)

Flaxseed oil (high lignan)

Macadamia oil (omega-7)

MCT oil

Olive oil, extra-virgin first cold-pressed

Perilla oil (lots of ALA and rosemarinic acid, both uncouplers)

Red palm oil (some effect)

Rice bran oil

Sesame oil, regular and toasted

Walnut oil (some effect)

Nuts and Seeds
Up to $^1/_2$ cup per day.

Almonds (only blanched or marcona)

Barùkas (or baru) nuts

Basil seeds

Brazil nuts (in limited quantities)

Chestnuts

Coconut meat (but not coconut water)

Coconut milk/cream (unsweetened full-fat canned)

Coconut milk (unsweetened dairy substitute)

Flaxseeds

Hazelnuts

Hemp protein powder

Hemp seeds

Macadamia nuts

Milkadamia creamer (unsweetened and not the milk)

Nut butters (if almond butter, preferably made with blanched almonds, as almond skins contain lectins)

Pecans

Pine nuts

Pili nuts

Pistachios

Psyllium seeds/psyllium husk powder

Sacha inchi seeds

Sesame seeds

Tahini

Walnuts

"Energy" Bars

Limit to one per day, please.

Adapt: coconut, chocolate (adaptyourlife.com)

Fast Bar

Gundry MD bars

Keto Bars: almond butter brownie, salted caramel, lemon poppy seed, chocolate chip cookie dough

KetoBars.com: mint chocolate, dark chocolate coconut almond, chocolate-covered strawberry

Keto Krisp: chocolate mint, almond butter, chocolate raspberry, almond butter chocolate chip, almond butter & blackberry jelly

Kiss My Keto: cookie dough, chocolate coconut, birthday cake

MariGold: ChocoNut, Pure Joy, espresso, ginger coconut

Primal Kitchen: almond spice, coconut lime

Rowdy Bars: keto chocolaty cookie dough

Stoka: vanilla almond, coco almond

Processed Resistant Starches

Can be eaten every day in limited quantities; those with prediabetes or diabetes should consume only once a week on average.

Barely Bread bread and bagels (only those without raisins)

Bread SRSLY sourdough non-lectin bread and rice-free sourdough rolls

Cappello's fettuccine and other pasta

Crepini egg thins

Fullove Foods keto hemp and linseed bread

Julian Bakery Paleo wraps (made with coconut flour), Paleo
thin bread, almond bread, sandwich bread, coconut bread

Lovebird Cereals (unsweetened only)

Mikey's original and toasted onion English muffins, cassava flour
tortillas

ONANA Tortillas

Positively Plantain tortillas

The Real Coconut coconut and cassava flour tortillas and chips

Siete chips (be careful here, a couple of my "canaries" react
to the small amount of chia seeds in the chips) and tortillas
(only those made with cassava and coconut flour or almond
flour)

Terra cassava, taro, and plantain chips

Thrive Market organic coconut flakes

Tia Lupita grain-free cactus tortillas

Trader Joe's jicama wraps, plantain chips

Uprising Food breads and crackers (Uprisingfood.com)

Resistant Starches

Eat in moderation. People with diabetes and prediabetes should initially limit these foods.

Baobab fruit

Cassava (tapioca)

Celery root (celeriac)

Glucomannan (konjac root)

Green bananas

Green mango

Green papaya

Green plantains

GundryMD Popped Superfood Crisps

Jicama

Millet

Parsnips

Persimmon

Rutabaga

Sorghum

Sweet potatoes or yams

Taro root

Tiger nuts

Turnips

Yucca

"Foodles" (acceptable "noodles")

Big Green millet and sorghum pastas

Edison Grainery sorghum pasta

Gundry MD sorghum spaghetti

Jovial cassava pastas

Kelp noodles

Konjac noodles

Miracle Noodle kanten pasta

Miracle Rice

Natural Heaven hearts of palm spaghetti and lasagna noodles

Palmini hearts of palm noodles

Shirataki noodles

Slimdown360 sweet potato pasta elbow macaroni

Trader Joe's cauliflower gnocchi

Wild-Caught Seafood

(4 ounces per day)

Alaskan salmon

Anchovies

Calamari/squid

Canned tuna

Clams

Cod

Crab

Freshwater bass

Halibut

Hawaiian fish, including mahimahi, ono, and opah

Lake Superior whitefish

Lobster

Mussels

Oysters

Sardines

Scallops

Shrimp (wild only)

Steelhead

Trout

Pastured Poultry
(*4 ounces per day*)

Chicken

Duck

Game birds (pheasant, grouse, dove, quail)

Goose

Ostrich

Pastured or omega-3 eggs (up to 4 daily)

Turkey

Meat
(*100 percent grass-fed and grass-finished; 4 ounces per day*)

Beef

Bison

Boar

Elk

Grass-fed jerky (low-sugar versions)

Lamb

Pork (humanely raised, including prosciutto, Ibérico ham, Cinco Jotas ham, Canadian bacon, ham)

Venison

Wild game

Plant-Based Proteins and "Meats"

Flaxseed protein powder

Gundry MD ProPlant protein shakes

Hemp protein powder

Hemp tofu

Hilary's root veggie burger (hilaryseatwell.com)

Perfect Day vegan whey and casein

Pressure-cooked lentils and other legumes (canned, such as Eden or Jovial brand) or dried, soaked, then pressure cooked (use an Instant Pot)

Protein isolates of and/or hydrolyzed pea, soy, or other similar bean powders (not the same as regular pea protein, soy protein, lentil protein, chickpea protein—buyer beware!)

Quorn products: only meatless pieces, meatless grounds, meatless steak-style strips, meatless fillets, meatless roast (avoid all others as they contain lectins/gluten)

Textured vegetable protein (TVP)

Vegg vegan egg yolks and products

Polyphenol-Rich Fruits

Limit to one small serving on weekends and only when that fruit is in season, or unlimited with "reverse juicing" (see page 123). Best options are pomegranate and passion fruit seeds, followed by raspberries, blackberries, strawberries, then blueberries, grapefruit, pixie tangerines, and kiwifruits (eat the skin for more polyphenols).

Apples

Apricots

Blackberries

Blueberries

Cherries

Citrus, all types (no juices)

Cranberries (fresh)

Guava

Kiwis

Nectarines

Papaya

Passion fruit

Peaches

Pears, crispy (Anjou, Bosc, Comice)

Persimmon

Plums

Pomegranates

Raspberries

Starfruit

Strawberries

Dairy Products and Replacements (top uncouplers)

Aged cheeses from Switzerland

Aged "raw" French/Italian cheeses

Buffalo butter (available at Trader Joe's)

Buffalo mozzarella: mozzarella di bufala (Italy), Buf Creamery (Uruguay)

Coconut yogurt (plain)

French/Italian butter

Ghee (grass-fed)

Goat and sheep kefir (plain)

Goat ghee

Goat milk cream flakes: Mt. Capra

Goat milk powder: Meyenberg, Hoosier Hill Farm, The Good
Goat Milk Company

Goat's-milk cheeses: feta, Brie, mozzarella, cheddar

Goat yogurt (plain)

Kite Hill Ricotta Cheese

Lavva plant-based yogurt

Organic cream cheese

Organic heavy cream

Organic sour cream

Parmigiano-Reggiano cheese

Sheep yogurt (plain)

Sheep's-milk cheeses: Pecorino Romano, Pecorino Sardo, feta,
Manchego

So Delicious Vegan Mozzarella, Cream Cheese

Herbs, Seasonings, and Condiments

Avocado mayonnaise

Coconut aminos

Fish sauce

Herbs and spices (all except red pepper flakes)

MCT mayonnaise

Miso paste

Mustard

Nutritional yeast

Pure vanilla extract

R's KOSO, Other KOSOs

Sea salt (iodized)

Tahini

Vinegars (apple cider vinegars, Bliss Vinegars, Sideyard Shrubs
Vinegars, others)

Wasabi

Flours

Almond (blanched, not almond meal)

Arrowroot

Cassava

Chestnut

Coconut

Coffee fruit

Grape seed

Green banana

Hazelnut

Millet

Sesame (and seeds)

Sorghum flour

Sweet potato

Tiger nut

Sweeteners

Allulose (look for non-GMO)

Erythritol (Swerve is my favorite, as it also contains oligosaccharides)

Inulin (Just Like Sugar is a great brand)

Local honey and/or manuka honey (very limited!)

Monk fruit (luo han guo; the Nutresse brand is good)

Stevia (SweetLeaf is my favorite; also contains inulin)

Xylitol

Yacon syrup (Super Yacon Syrup is available at Walmart; Sunfood Sweet Yacon Syrup is available on Amazon)

Chocolate and Frozen Desserts

Coconut milk dairy-free frozen desserts (the So Delicious blue label, which contains only 1 gram of sugar; but be careful: may contain pea protein)

Dark chocolate, unsweetened, 72% cacao or greater (1 ounce per day)

Enlightened ice cream

Keto Ice Cream: chocolate, mint chip, sea salt caramel

Killer Creamery ice cream: Chilla in Vanilla, Caramels Back, and No Judge Mint

Mammoth Creameries: vanilla bean

Natural (non-Dutched) cocoa powder, unsweetened

Nick's vegan ice cream

Rebel Creamery ice cream: butter pecan, raspberry, salted caramel, strawberry, vanilla

Simple Truth ice cream: butter pecan and chocolate chip

Beverages

Champagne (6 ounces per day)

Coffee

Dark spirits (1 ounce per day)

Hydrogen water

KeVita brand low-sugar kombucha (coconut, coconut Mojito, for example), other low-sugar kombuchas

San Pellegrino or Acqua Panna water

Red wine (6 ounces per day)

Tea (all types)

No, Thank You: Major Lectin-Containing Foods

Refined, Starchy Foods

Bread

Cereal

Cookies

Crackers

Pasta

Pastries

Potato chips

Potatoes

Rice

Tortillas

Wheat flour

Grains, Sprouted Grains, Pseudograins, and Grasses

Barley (cannot pressure cook)

Barley grass

Brown rice

Buckwheat

Bulgur

Corn

Corn products

Corn syrup

Einkorn

Kamut

Kasha

Oats (cannot pressure cook)

Popcorn

Quinoa

Rye (cannot pressure cook)

Spelt

Wheat (pressure cooking does not remove lectins from any form of wheat)

Wheatgrass

White rice (except pressure cooked white basmati rice from

India, which is high resistant starch; American white basmati is not)

Wild rice

Sugar and Sweeteners

Agave

Coconut sugar

Diet drinks

Granulated sugar (even organic cane sugar)

Maltodextrin

NutraSweet (aspartame)

Splenda (sucralose; Splenda now has an allulose product that is acceptable; see page 153)

Sweet One and Sunett (acesulfame-K)

Sweet'N Low (saccharin)

Vegetables
Most of these can be made safe foods with
pressure cooking; marked with an (*).

All beans* (including sprouts)

Chickpeas* (including as hummus)

Edamame*

Green/string beans*

Legumes*

All lentils*

Pea protein (unless pea protein isolate or hydrolysate)

Peas*

Soy*

Soy protein (unless soy protein isolate or hydrolysate)

Sugar snap peas

Tofu*

Nuts and Seeds

Almonds, unblanched

Cashews

Chia seeds

Peanuts

Pumpkin seeds

Sunflower seeds

Fruits

(some we call vegetables)

Bell peppers

Chile peppers

Cucumbers

Eggplant

Goji berries

Melons (any kind)

Pumpkins

Squash (any kind)

Tomatillos

Tomatoes

Zucchini

Milk Products that Contain A1 Beta-Casein

Butter (even grass-fed), unless from A2 cows, sheep, or goats, or buffalo

Cheese

Cottage cheese

Cow's milk

Frozen yogurt

Ice cream (most)

Kefir from American cows

Ricotta

Yogurt (including Greek yogurt)

Oils

All "partially hydrogenated" oils

Corn

Cottonseed

Grapeseed

Peanut

Safflower

Soy

Sunflower

"Vegetable"

Herbs and Seasonings

Ketchup

Mayonnaise (unless MCT or avocado)

Red pepper flakes

Soy sauce

Steak sauce

Worcestershire sauce

These dos and don'ts provide the foundation for you to harness the power of mitochondrial uncoupling, this heretofore little-known process that is the secret to good health and long life. When you follow these guidelines, you have the power to upregulate your uncoupling gene activity by making or consuming ketones, liberating free fatty acids from your fat stores, and consuming foods that give your microbiome access to short-chain fatty acids, postbiotics, and polyphenols.

For too long, we've been talking about healthy eating in terms of antioxidant-rich and fibrous foods. But you now understand that these are just code words for what's really behind health and longevity: polyphenols and postbiotic-producing foods, all of which deliver their desirable effects by uncoupling your mitochondria. In fact, the next time someone tells you to "eat the rainbow," know that it really means "eat to uncouple."

CHAPTER 10

MOVING TOWARD KETO-CONSUMPTION

Unlocking the keto code isn't just about the foods you eat (and don't eat!)—you also need to consider *when* you should eat. Recently, the once niche practice of time-controlled eating, sometimes called intermittent fasting, has gained widespread appeal. These days, it seems you can't open a magazine or look at a health-related article on the internet without a mention of intermittent fasting or time-controlled eating.

In my last book, *The Energy Paradox*, I introduced a new approach to time-restricted eating that I called chrono-consumption. In this book, I refine that approach to bring you keto-consumption! Not only does this timed eating plan help boost energy, but more important, it increases the production of ketones and other powerful signaling compounds that uncouple mitochondria. This decisive schedule is strategically timed to maximize your mitochondria's rest and repair functions, helping you phase in and out of ketosis in ways that will boost your health and longevity. But asking you to immediately jump from your current eating habits and schedule to where you should be in five weeks is quite a bit to ask. So this program, like its predecessor, chrono-consumption, will ease you into the kind of eating schedule that promotes the making of ketones. It's a great way to slowly transition to time-controlled eating (intermittent fasting) without too much fuss or frustration. And now, thanks to feedback from my patients and you, dear readers, I've made making the switch to time-controlled eating even easier so you can get the most out of keto-consumption!

After all, I understand that for many people, increasing the wait time between the last meal of one day and the first meal of the next is the most challenging part of unlocking the keto code. To start, no one likes to be hungry. But on top of that, starting as early as grade school, Big Food has told us that breakfast is essential—they even say you can't start your day without it! It can be tough to shake that mind-set, and tougher still to start the day on an empty stomach. Never fear: the Keto Code program will help you slowly build up to keto-consumption's recommended eating window. Before you know it, you'll easily wake up in the morning and fast until noon without even thinking about it. (And if you *are* thinking about it, we'll set you up with some simple hacks that will fool your body into continuing to make ketones even as you eat.)

I've learned a lot from my patients and readers since the release of *The Energy Paradox*. Those who adopted the chrono-consumption program shared what worked for them and what was challenging, and based on their feedback, I've simplified my recommendations.

We'll start off by easing into things. There's no need to bite off more than you can chew, if you'll excuse the pun. Instead of trying to jump into an 18-hour fast, which, believe it or not, will become easy in just a few weeks' time, we'll begin with a shorter eating window (the amount of time you can eat in any 24-hour period) of 12 hours and work our way down from there. Week by week over the next five weeks, you'll shorten that window to 6 to 8 hours each day, if possible, while also abstaining from food for at least 3 hours before bedtime. Doing so will give your body, your mitochondria, your gut buddies, and your brain the time they need to rest, repair, and regenerate.

Reading this, you may still think it's impossible. I assure you, it is not! Thousands of my patients have succeeded in adopting a time-controlled eating program over the past few years. But as an extra incentive, I'll add this: you will only need to maintain this compressed eating window Monday through Friday. As a reward for taking care of your mitochondria during the week, you can eat as you like on weekends—no eating window required! You're going to be embracing the keto-consumption lifestyle before you know it.

Slowly compressing the period of time during which you eat helps your body become metabolically flexible. I've had over twenty years of experience working with insulin-resistant, prediabetic, and diabetic patients. I've witnessed them struggle with traditional keto-style diets, year after year. Remember: If you're insulin resistant, your mitochondria likely can't switch from burning glucose (carbs) to burning free fatty acids (FFAs) to make ATP. And even if they could, having a high insulin level prevents your fat cells from releasing FFAs. If you can't release FFAs from the body's fat cells, you can't generate uncoupling ketones. That means you're basically set up to fail on most ketogenetic diet plans, no matter how many carbs you cut or how much fat you eat.

So let's talk more about what keto-consumption entails and how you can use it to upgrade your health. Rather than jumping into the deep end, we're going to slowly and carefully wade into the baby pool to help our mitochondria get rested, repaired, and ready to uncouple!

CRACKING THE KETO CODE THROUGH KETO-CONSUMPTION

To help facilitate mitochondrial uncoupling, you want to make ketones as well as release FFAs from your fat cells. Remember, to start making ketones and mobilize those fats, you need at least 12 hours during which you don't consume any calories. I've created the following keto-consumption schedule to ease you into the program. Each week is broken down as follows:

- **Week 1:** On week 1 of keto-consumption, you'll start breakfast at eight a.m. and finish your last meal of the day by seven p.m., Monday through Friday. Once the weekend comes around, you can be more flexible (within reason!). You can eat your breakfast when you like, maybe even sharing the meal with friends and family, provided you're still following the Keto Code program's eating dos and don'ts and list of approved foods.
- **Week 2:** Week 2 is much like week 1, except this week, delay your first meal of the day by one hour, breaking your fast at nine a.m.
- **Weeks 3 through 5:** Each successive week, you'll follow the same basic schedule, but you'll push breakfast up by another hour each week. During week 3, breakfast is at ten a.m. Week 4? Eleven a.m. And so on and so forth, until you don't have your first bite until noon, condensing your daily eating window to a mere 7 hours (noon to seven p.m.).

Note: I default to seven p.m. as the end of the day's eating window, as that seems to work best for most of my patients. It allows them to have dinner around the time they prefer to eat, while also giving them the space to have that 3-hour break before bedtime.

But the eating windows I've mentioned here are not absolute. You may have different needs due to a specific work schedule or your family commitments. It doesn't matter if you break your fast at nine a.m. and stop eating at four p.m. The idea here is that you gradually ease your way into a 6- to 8-hour eating window to maximize ketone production and release those FFAs so your mitochondria will get to uncoupling.

For some—especially those who've never loved eating breakfast—transitioning to a restricted eating window is relatively painless. But most people need a more staggered approach to be successful (and, I might add, all my patients who have followed this schedule have been!). By pushing breakfast back gradually and loosening the reins a bit on the weekends, you'll find the process of shortening your eating window to be easier on both the body and the mind. It's not unlike trying a new fitness routine. No one expects you to hop off the couch and finish a marathon without training, or to hold a plank for 10 minutes your first time out the gate. You work up to it over time. Similarly, when it comes to keto-consumption, you'll train to embrace a smaller eating window over five weeks. You'll find this is a

THE BASIC KETO-CONSUMPTION EATING SCHEDULE

WEEK	Monday Breakfast	Tuesday Breakfast	Wednesday Breakfast	Thursday Breakfast	Friday Breakfast
1	*8A.M.	8 A.M.	8 A.M.	8 A.M.	8 A.M.
2	9 A.M.	9 A.M.	9 A.M.	9 A.M.	9 A.M.
3	10 A.M.	10 A.M.	10 A.M.	10 A.M.	10 A.M.
4	11 A.M.	11 A.M.	11 A.M.	11 A.M.	11 A.M.
5	12 P.M.	12 P.M.	12 P.M.	12 P.M.	12 P.M.

proven schedule that will allow you to become more metabolically flexible—and get those mitochondria uncoupling—without muss or fuss. And once you've made it through the first five weeks, enjoying those more flexible weekends along the way, you'll quickly see that keto-consumption is an eating style that can work with just about any lifestyle. This has not only been my experience, but is supported by studies that show such a schedule helps to support compliance without interfering with an individual's metabolic flexibility.[1]

Once you complete the initial five-week keto-consumption schedule, you may notice some changes. To start, your metabolism will now be in a state where it can waste fat more easily. And you'll be making ketones without having to consume all that unappetizing fat! Between the released FFAs and the ketones, your mitochondria will be receiving all the signals they need to start uncoupling, repair themselves, and increase their numbers throughout the cells in your body. Even better? You'll have become accustomed to your condensed eating window. Keeping the keto-consumption schedule won't seem like a hardship anymore. Once week 6 rolls around, you'll stick with the program without reservation. By week 10, you'll love the results so much that you won't remember why you ate the way you did before! It may take some time, but before you know it, you'll have adopted a wonderful new eating style that will improve your health, well-being, and longevity. (And yes, help you lose those unwanted pounds, too!)

Uncoupling Beverages

Just because you're limiting your eating window doesn't mean you need to limit how much fluid you consume during the day. In fact, staying hydrated makes it easier to ease your way into keto-consumption. When you're getting enough to drink, you feel less hungry.

I recommend drinking filtered water to eliminate any water-borne toxins. But if you have a choice of waters, my go-to is San Pellegrino sparkling water. Not only is it pH balanced, it also has the highest purity and sulfur content of any bottled water on the market. (Also, the CO_2 that provides the bubbles may benefit blood flow to your organs and brain.) To give your water a little extra oomph, try adding a dash of balsamic or apple cider vinegar to make a refreshing sparkler. You'll get an extra dose of polyphenols and short-chain fatty acids (SCFAs), allowing you to simultaneously hydrate and uncouple!

Remember, when choosing a beverage, if there is an uncoupler and/or polyphenol present, so much the better. That means you should feel free to indulge your morning caffeine habit. You can have tea—either green or black—or black coffee. All these beverages are rich in polyphenols (and, contrary to popular belief, they don't dehydrate you). Remember, caffeine works as a mitochondrial uncoupler in its own right! Afraid of caffeine? Get the decaf varieties or have an herbal tea made with uncouplers like mint. And if you aren't ready to give up your creamer just yet, choose one of the many keto MCT creamers on the market.

I'm sure you also have questions about alcohol. For women, I recommend consuming no more than 4 to 6 ounces of organic or biodynamic red wine or champagne with dinner; for men, double that. If you prefer spirits, you can have 1 ounce of your favorite dark spirit during your evening meal. Why dark spirits and not clear alcohol like vodka or gin? Dark spirits have been aged in wood casks, and in the process, they've absorbed uncoupling polyphenols from the wood itself! Why red wine and not white? Studies show dramatic improvements in the gut buddies and inflammation markers of red wine drinkers versus clear spirits.[2]

JUST SAY NO (TO A MEAL)

From a young age, we're told that we need to eat three square meals a day—plus a couple of snacks. That is decidedly not the case, and it's often easier to move to a keto-consumption schedule by just saying no to lunch. Admittedly, skipping meals is not the easiest habit to pick up. After all, our modern lifestyles have us very accustomed to eating whenever and wherever we want. That said, it is far from impossible to skip a meal, or even two.

As you start to condense your eating window, you may feel some hunger—and let's face it, no one likes being hungry. The first two weeks of this program can be a little challenging if you're used to eating first thing in the morning. Having said that, feeling hungry is normal—and you're experiencing those feelings because your body is not yet metabolically flexible enough to switch over to fat-burning mode. When you stick with the program long enough to start reaping its many benefits, your metabolism will start getting the right messages from your microbiome and mitochondria, diminishing those hunger pangs in the process. But if you're finding it hard to stick with the program, here are a few tips to help manage your hunger:

Have some MCT oil. Have a spoonful of MCT oil (preferably the C8 or C10 varieties, which are more ketogenic) three times a day. You can start with a teaspoon to help you get through those sinking spells, and eventually move up to a tablespoon. A note of caution, however: Some people experience some gastrointestinal distress after ingesting MCT oil. This is common in many of my female patients.

I recommend using it sparingly at first and working your way up to larger amounts. Some people do much better with MCT powders, several of which are available as coffee creamers. The beauty of MCT oil is that it will not break your fast—and as a bonus, it will signal your liver to start making ketones, even if your fasting insulin level is initially high and you can't liberate FFAs from your fat cells to make ketones the old-fashioned way just yet.

Slow the pace. Okay, so maybe week 1 was a piece of cake (pardon the pun), but now that week 2 has rolled around, you feel hungry, cranky, and completely devoid of energy as you try to wait until nine a.m. to eat. That little inner voice says there's no way you'll make it till nine! If you managed breakfast at eight a.m. without issue, stay there for week 2, then try for eight thirty or nine a.m. the next week. Each week, set a new goal for pushing back breakfast. It may take you more than five weeks, but you'll get there, slowly but surely! And don't forget: Worst-case scenario, you can have one of the approved keto bars from the "Yes, Please" foods list (most of which contain uncoupling MCTs) to get you through to breakfast. I'll have more to say on this trick in just a moment.

Eat the right foods. One of the best ways to keep hunger pangs at bay is to increase the amount of prebiotic fiber or fermented foods you ingest. You can add it to your meals, but I find the best way is to just mix a scoop of prebiotic fiber powder into some water and drink it. Because you can't digest it, it doesn't break your fast, but it's the best breakfast your gut buddies could ever ask for. They'll send messages via postbiotics to tell your brain they are content and no more food is required. (They'll start producing butyrate, that incredible mitochondrial fuel and uncoupler, to boot.)

Add some vinegar. You can quell hunger pangs by adding a little vinegar to a glass of water. I generally put about 2 tablespoons of balsamic or apple cider vinegar in my glass of San Pellegrino first thing in the morning or whenever I experience a hungry feeling. The post-biotics and SCFAs in these vinegars have the power to kick-start mitochondrial uncoupling from the very first swallow. And not only will they not break your fast, but they'll also enhance mitochondrial uncoupling even more because of their postbiotics.

Enjoy an MCT Capraccino. No, that's not a typo for "cappuccino"! I use the term "capraccino" to refer to the Latin *capra* for the genus of goat. This tasty beverage will increase ketone production and uncoupling; see page 183 for the recipe.

Eat MCT-rich goat, sheep, and water buffalo dairy products as your first meal. Remember, any time you can harness the power of MCTs to kick-start the production of ketones by the liver—especially early in the program—the better off you'll be. While many people have no issues with MCT liquids or powders, some may experience gastrointestinal issues like diarrhea or nausea. That's where goat, sheep, and water buffalo cheeses and yogurts can make a big difference. These milk products are composed of about 30 percent MCTs—so it becomes an extremely tasty and ketogenic way to start the day without having to extend your fasting hours.

Keep nuts nearby. Whenever a hunger pang feels unbearable, eat 1 ounce of nuts (that works out to be about a generous handful.) Salted nuts are best for this. I buy most nuts raw—I buy barùkas (or baru) nuts and sacha inchi seeds, which have a high polyphenol content, roasted—and then grind iodized sea salt onto them in my palm. When you are actively losing weight, you urinate more frequently—and in the process, you lose sodium. Research shows that it is beneficial to increase your salt intake as you work to shorten your eating window. While most health experts have made salt out to be a nutritional bad guy, it's not the enemy everyone seems to think it is. Ketones actually compete with uric acid (the mischief maker that causes gout) to be excreted from the kidneys. But you can solve this problem by increasing your salt consumption by about a teaspoon a day. Just make sure it's iodized sea salt, as the pink stuff or other varieties of sea salt you may find on grocery store shelves does not contain iodine.

I'd add that I'm also fond of electrolyte replacement powders like those made by the brand LMNT. We even have our own version at Gundry MD. That said, I recommend avoiding most popular electrolyte drinks, even the sugar-free ones, as they tend to be loaded with toxic artificial sweeteners that will destroy your gut microbiome.

Eat a nut or coconut bar. In exciting research published in 2021, my friend and colleague Dr. Valter Longo at the University of Southern California reported that eating a 200-calorie, mostly nut-based bar called a Fast Bar did *not* interrupt ketone production or raise blood sugar in people who were following a time-restricted eating plan like you will being doing in the Keto Code program. You heard that right—eating this kind of bar did *not* interrupt their ketone production from an overnight fast![3] This is good news. It means that a handful of nuts or a nut-based bar will not sabotage your ketone-generating efforts (see page 142 for a list of approved bars). And it will probably keep the hunger demon at bay, too.

Take ketones directly. Another option to help you deal with your hunger as you adopt the Keto Code program and start to make your own ketones is to take a few capsules or a scoop of preformed ketones in the form of ketone salts or esters. Believe it or not, these supplements are the real deal—and quickly tell your mitochondria it's time to start uncoupling. As you learned in earlier chapters, ingested ketones have the same beneficial effects on changing the gut microbiome as the traditional ketogenic diet. While ketone salts are relatively easy to find, the esters, quite frankly, are very expensive and taste pretty terrible. For my money (and yours), stick with MCT oils or goat's- and sheep's-milk products.

Have breakfast early. Finally, on some days, you may be struggling and psychologically need to feel fueled and alert. Maybe you have a big presentation or an extra-hard workout. In these cases, have your breakfast a bit early—or grab one of those nut bars on your way out the door. The next day, you can get right back on track.

Any time you make changes to your diet and lifestyle, it is common to experience challenges and setbacks. No matter what, go easy on yourself and do your best to stay the course.

GIVING UP GRAZING

Sadly, the average American doesn't limit themselves to just three meals a day. Rather, they graze all day long. In fact, the latest research suggests the average human eats for 16 hours of the day!

In some ways, that's understandable. Modern life is busy—and these days, we're all at home a lot more often than we used to be, with a million opportunities to walk by the kitchen and peer into the fridge. It's easy to take a small bite here, a little nosh there, regardless of the time of day. When patients come to see me for the first time, most have never had their fasting insulin level measured before. Much like Miranda, they share their stories about failed attempts at traditional ketogenic diets or intermittent fasting. They blame themselves for their dietary failures, but the reality is, they never stood a chance of success because they're eating all the time. They simply didn't have the mitochondrial flexibility to use FFAs in the way they were designed to be used. But when you slowly taper off sugar and eliminate all those unnecessary mini meals, your body will quickly learn how to use fat for fuel and make ketones, which will signal uncoupling and mitogenesis and mitochondrial repair.

Now, some of you may be thinking, "Look, I'm not one of your usual patients, Dr. G. I eat only healthy, organic food!" Or maybe you're insistent that you already eat a perfect keto diet: "No dirty keto, no protein-sparing keto, I'm locked in at eighty percent fat, Doc. But I'm still overweight. What about me?" Well, I have a few things to say about both cases.

First, most of you so-called healthy eaters are still consuming a smorgasbord of lectin-rich foods that are destroying your gut wall, producing inflammation. So many of my new patients are just like Miranda, who, remember, was apoplectic that she had high insulin levels despite two years of "keto" commitment. Miranda was eating lectin-containing cheese products, and those lectins were enough to throw her gut wall into disrepair. Moreover, her cow's-milk cheeses had none of the beneficial MCTs found in goat's- and sheep's-milk cheeses. Her mitochondria weren't getting all the signals they needed to take care of themselves, and as a result, her overall health suffered. In addition, most of you "perfect keto" people aren't getting any plant polyphenols and fibers to kick-start mitochondrial uncoupling.

Also, remember those mice who munched all day on their healthy rat chow? Despite that healthy food, they still didn't have any metabolic flexibility. If you're eating healthily or even high-fat keto, but you're eating constantly over a long window each day, you're still setting yourself up for failure. You need to limit your eating hours to fully harness keto-consumption.

Finally, many of my self-described healthy eaters are downright addicted to fruit when they first meet me. Remember, nature's candies get their sweetness from energy-robbing fructose. Too much of it will overwhelm your liver and mitochondria.[4]

If you're reading this and see that your current diet contains some of these keto-consumption faux pas, don't be discouraged. Even after your first couple of weeks on this program—your proverbial baby steps into greater mitochondrial health and uncoupling—you'll start to notice a real difference in your overall well-being. And once you start to feel those effects, you will, no doubt, be motivated to keep going.

Embracing Some Flexibility

While I've offered a basic schedule for keto-consumption, one of the biggest benefits of this form of time-controlled eating is that it offers some flexibility. Provided you strive for a shortened eating window, you can schedule your meals as best fits your lifestyle.

For example, I have patients who are stubbornly attached to having breakfast at a certain time in the morning. They feel they need to start the day with something in their belly or they simply cannot (or will not—I'm not entirely certain which is more accurate) function for the rest of the day. Those people (you know who you are) have two options: you can always grab a nut bar that won't interrupt ketone creation, as I mentioned earlier; or you can go for what I like to call the Ramadan option.

If you're familiar with the Islamic faith, you likely know that the ninth month of the Islamic calendar is called Ramadan. During this time, tradition dictates that devout Muslims fast from dawn to sunset and pray. Most families eat a small breakfast before the sun rises and then abstain from food or drink until after sunset. That evening meal tends to be the main meal of the day, where families feast together in celebration.

I mention this because this type of eating schedule can also offer a condensed eating window. By fasting for 12 hours during the day and then again for 8 hours overnight, those who follow Ramadan traditions are essentially fasting—and making ketones, releasing FFAs, and telling their mitochondria to uncouple—for 20 hours across a 24-hour period!

That said, while this approach works for some people as opposed to the more traditional keto-consumption schedule, most studies show it doesn't promote weight loss. I've actually seen this firsthand in my own patients. They get most of the health benefits associated with time-controlled eating—we see a drop in insulin levels and an improvement in blood work—but about half the people who follow this type of schedule don't lose any weight. As I review these patients' food diaries, I've noticed a trend in the people who maintain their weight: they tend to indulge in a huge meal at night, supplemented with generous portions of dried fruits like figs and dates. That likely explains why those extra pounds stay put!

Despite the fact that not everyone will lose weight using the Ramadan approach, there are still benefits to trying this option if you are stuck fast (see what I did there?) on eating a more traditional breakfast.

If you find yourself struggling on the keto-consumption schedule—and I mean this sincerely—I don't want to lose you and your mitochondria because it's too hard to compress your eating window. Try eating breakfast, skip lunch, and then wait for dinner as your last meal of the day. Even better, grab a handful of nuts, a piece of goat's- or sheep's-milk cheese, or an approved bar for your breakfast. It's likely that in time, as your metabolism adjusts and becomes more flexible, you'll find you're more than ready to start pushing out your breakfast to a later hour.

(Also, for those of you who have advanced on the keto-consumption path and want to keep up your progress on the weekends, you could try the Ramadan option on Saturdays and Sundays. That is actually what I do almost every weekend throughout the year.)

Another option that some of my patients appreciate is the one-meal-a-day (OMAD) plan. This approach has the power to turbo boost the Keto Code plan and really rev up your metabolism. If you're already engaging in some form of intermittent fasting—or just found the first five weeks of the schedule fairly easy—you can step up your uncoupling power by eating only a single meal each day.

This is how I conduct my own time-restricted eating for a large part of each year. From January to June, I eat just a single meal sometime between six p.m. and eight p.m. That's right: I fast 22 hours a day, five days a week, six months of the year. While this option may seem extreme (and many of you may doubt it is even possible!), I can assure you that it is not only possible but, with time, easier to sustain than you might think.

And the results are undeniable! When my patients try the OMAD approach to keto-consumption, you can immediately see the difference in their blood work. Their IGF-1 levels drop, their HbA1C improves, and their overall health blossoms. It's mitochondrial uncoupling in action! By significantly reducing the time your gut spends digesting food, you can give your mitochondria the rest they need to uncouple and thrive.

If you're wondering why I don't indulge in OMAD year-round, you can chalk it up to our ancestors. Our hunter-gatherer forebears had to cope with limited food during the winter and spring. Summer and fall, of course, brought bountiful options. By taking this more seasonal approach, which is deeply engrained in our genes, your mitochondria will benefit. This is the Goldilocks Rule in action—when you cycle between ketosis and a sated state, your mitochondria can better flourish.

While this may seem like a rather extreme ketogenic state—and it's not for everyone—it can be done. If you'd like to give it a try, I suggest starting after the five-week marker, when you're eating your first meal at noon and stopping all food intake by seven p.m. During week 6, you can push your first meal to one p.m. Week 7, two p.m. And so on and so forth until you reach the two-hour OMAD window by week 11.

If you are considering going OMAD, I must also offer a word of caution. Over and over again, I and others have shown how continuous ketosis is unhealthy. Never in the history of mankind have humans thrived by starving themselves over the long term. Our bodies are designed to manage feast and famine. But famine on its own? That's a nonstarter. So, if you go OMAD, again, lighten up on the weekend and have two meals a day, maybe even three.

I mention the Ramadan and OMAD options to, once again, illustrate that there are many ways to successfully embrace keto-consumption. Provided you aim for a condensed eating window, you can find a schedule that will uncouple your mitochondria in a manner that works for you, your needs, and your lifestyle.

The Skinny on Macros and Calories

What about them? Unlike many popular diets and eating plans, you don't have to worry about counting calories or tracking macronutrients on the Keto Code program. I'm not joking! You're free to leave all that behind. I highly recommend that you do so. In fact, to date, I have never put a calorie count or protein/fat/carb breakdown in any of my recipes—and for good reason. You don't need to worry about it.

We are learning that calorie counts don't mean much at all,

particularly if a lot of those calories are being eaten by your gut buddies as they produce postbiotics. And frankly, I'm not concerned with your ratios of protein, fat, and carbs. For emphasis, let me repeat that: I'm not concerned about you eating huge amounts of fats to get into ketosis. I'm not worried about you limiting your carbohydrate intake—in fact, I want you to eat all the polyphenols you can! And as you've learned in the earlier chapters of this book, there's no need for you to put such restrictions on your diet. Study after study has shown that time-restricted eating works better than calorie restriction to fix metabolic flexibility.[5] So follow your keto-consumption schedule, eat your fill of "Yes, Please" foods, and enjoy!

Truly, your ultimate health and longevity do not depend on limiting calories or some complicated dance of balancing out a particular ratio of macronutrients. Rather, your overall well-being depends on being able to uncouple your mitochondria so they can not only survive, but thrive! Just like Dr. de Cabo's mice, it doesn't matter what you eat (although you'll soon see that following the Keto Code plan's dos and don'ts will help you gain the metabolic flexibility you need to be successful). Rather, what matters most is when you eat, and for how long. By limiting your eating window and consuming foods that feed your gut buddies, you'll reap all the benefits of mitochondrial uncoupling—which you'll see as the numbers drop on the scale and feel in terms of overall health and well-being.

Okay, you now have the keto-consumption schedule to go with your eating dos and don'ts. By following the Keto Code plan, you'll set up your mitochondria for uncoupling and all its many benefits. Just follow the "Yes, Please" and "No, Thank You" foods lists (see Chapter 9) when making your meals and choosing your bars and snacks. I've also provided some new and exciting recipes for you to try in chapter 11, all of which incorporate uncoupling compounds in every delicious bite.

For too long, we've been talking about healthy eating in the wrong way. But you now understand what's really behind health and longevity. You want to eat polyphenols and postbiotic-producing foods, all of which deliver their desirable effects by uncoupling your mitochondria. That's why, every time someone says it's important to "eat the rainbow," what they are really saying is "eat to uncouple." You want to embrace keto-consumption and limit your eating window to 6 to 8 hours a day to produce ketones and release FFAs to help keep your mitochondria in tip-top shape. By doing so, you'll become an incredibly inefficient but remarkably healthy energy producer. What could be better than that?

By now, many of you are wondering what happened to poor Miranda, the keto failure you met earlier. Miranda, I'm pleased to say, has unlocked her mitochondria, is no longer insulin resistant, is no longer diabetic, and is fitting into new, smaller clothes. Even better, she feels great and is now eating great, once she learned these keys to unlock the keto code. Now it's your turn!

CHAPTER 11

THE KETO CODE RECIPES

Developing new recipes for a new program is one of my favorite projects, primarily because I get to experiment with new foods, flavors, and textures that I may not have explored before. With each new book, it is exciting to be able to introduce new foods that may be of benefit to a previously neglected aspect of your health.

Here in the Keto Code program, my goal is to highlight the delicious ways you can add flavorful uncoupling compounds to your everyday meals. In the following recipes, you'll see more fermented foods creatively (and deliciously) incorporated into fantastic dishes. After all, fermented foods offer huge health benefits. Not only do the probiotics they contain promote a more robust and diverse microbiome, but more important, fermented foods contain postbiotics like SCFAs and are the foods that allow your gut buddies to produce uncoupling postbiotics.

You will also notice that goat's- and sheep's-milk cheeses are at the forefront of many dishes. Remember, the MCTs in these cheeses are made into ketones in your liver, regardless of what else you may be eating, including carbs! But let's not forget to give aged, grass-fed, A2 cow's-milk cheeses from France, Italy, and Switzerland some love for all the uncoupling polyamines they contain, too. You should never hesitate to enjoy a simple plate of goat's-, sheep's-, or aged cow's-milk cheeses, as so many do in Europe, for your breakfast. (But unless you are eating approved breads, crackers, or tortillas from the Keto Code's "Yes, Please" foods list on page 142, you don't need to pair your cheese with crackers.)

It was also a lot of fun turning disastrous comfort foods (which, let's face it, aren't called "comfort foods" for nothing) like biscuits and gravy and spice cake into healthier dishes that are the definition of satisfaction and decadence. And I haven't forgotten my vegetarian and vegan readers. There are options to make these dishes just the way you want them—no animal protein or fats required.

Happy cooking and eating!

Uncoupling Capraccino

I know many of you can't start the day without your morning cup of java. Heck, I'm one of you! Here's my take on keto coffee, Uncoupling Capraccino. And no, that's not a typo! This drink harnesses the additional MCTs in goat's milk, cream, or cheese (hence the name, a play on *capra*, Latin for the genus that goats belong to and *cappuccino*), to give you a creamy, delicious beverage. This tasty pick-me-up will give you that little extra oomph through all of its uncoupling power!

For additional uncoupling power, add cinnamon, nutmeg, unsweetened natural (non-Dutched) cocoa powder, or cardamom as desired. The allulose or Just Like Sugar adds an extra boost of prebiotics.

Serves 1

1 cup hot coffee
1 tablespoon MCT oil
1 scoop powdered goat milk or goat cream (about 2 tablespoons), or
    1 ounce goat cheese or butter
Allulose, Just Like Sugar, monk fruit, or stevia

Combine all the ingredients in a blender and blend until frothy, about 30 seconds. Serve in a cup or mug.

Tropical Basil Seed Pudding

This pudding is perfect for anyone who loves chia seed pudding or rice pudding, but wants to enjoy it without the lectins. It's like a tropical vacation in a bowl—the combination of coconut, kiwi, and tangy passion fruit feels like an indulgent dessert, but you can enjoy this for breakfast or a snack anytime.

Serves 4

2 cups unsweetened full-fat coconut milk

2 tablespoons 1-for-1 monk fruit sweetener (such as Lakanto)

$^{1}/_{2}$ teaspoon pure vanilla extract

$^{1}/_{4}$ teaspoon pure coconut extract

$^{1}/_{4}$ cup basil seeds

$^{1}/_{2}$ cup unsweetened coconut flakes, toasted

1 kiwifruit, skin on, diced

$^{1}/_{2}$ cup fresh or unsweetened frozen passion fruit puree (from 3 or 4 passion fruit, if fresh)

1. In a large saucepan, combine the coconut milk and monk fruit and heat over medium heat, stirring occasionally, until the monk fruit has dissolved. Remove from the heat.
2. Add the vanilla, coconut extract, basil seeds, and half the coconut flakes and stir. Let stand for 5 minutes to allow the seeds to absorb the liquid.
3. Stir well, then transfer to four individual serving dishes and refrigerate for at least 3 to 4 hours to set.
4. In a small bowl, toss together the kiwi and passion fruit puree, then divide the fruit among the puddings. Top with the remaining coconut flakes just before serving.

Chocolate Coconut Smoothie

You may scan the ingredients below and think, "Cauliflower in a smoothie?!" Well, you won't taste it, but the frozen cauliflower rice gives this smoothie a texture that's similar to a fast-food milkshake. I like the subtle hint of anti-inflammatory cinnamon, but you can skip it if you want a more classic chocolate shake flavor.

Serves 1

1 cup unsweetened full-fat coconut milk
$^1/_2$ cup frozen cauliflower rice
2 tablespoons unsweetened cocoa powder
$^1/_2$ teaspoon pure vanilla extract
$^1/_4$ teaspoon ground cinnamon
1 teaspoon MCT oil
About 2 tablespoons 1-for-1 allulose or monk fruit sweetener

1. In a blender, combine the coconut milk, cauliflower rice, cocoa powder, vanilla, cinnamon, MCT oil, and one-third of the sweetener.
2. Blend until smooth, then taste and add more of the sweetener as needed.
3. Thin the milkshake with water until you can sip it through a straw, then enjoy.

Spicy Manchego Muffins

This recipe is a variation on one of the most popular recipes from my first cookbook—my cheesy cauliflower muffins, which a television host said reminded them of a popular seafood chain restaurant's biscuits. Don't skip the rosemary—it really adds something to this recipe.

Makes 12 muffins

3 cups cauliflower rice

3 omega-3 or pastured eggs or vegan egg substitute

$1/_2$ cup grated Manchego cheese or nutritional yeast

$1/_4$ cup almond flour

$1/_2$ teaspoon aluminum-free baking powder

1 teaspoon Old Bay seasoning

1 tablespoon minced fresh rosemary

Dash of hot sauce (optional)

1. Preheat the oven to 375°F. Line a standard muffin tin with paper liners.
2. In a large bowl, combine the cauliflower rice, eggs, and cheese.
3. In a small bowl, whisk together the almond flour, baking powder, and Old Bay.
4. Fold the dry ingredients into the cauliflower mixture along with the rosemary and hot sauce (if using), then portion the batter into the prepared muffin tin.
5. Bake for 20 to 25 minutes, until the tops of the muffins are no longer wet to the touch. Let cool for at least 5 minutes before serving.

Keto Biscuits and Gravy

This healthy twist on a diner-breakfast classic is great for a brunch with friends, or even a solo dinner. You can also make the biscuits on their own for when you want a dinner roll on the side of a meal. If you can't find xanthan gum, you can make the biscuits without it; they'll have a more crumbly texture.

Makes 12 biscuits

FOR THE BISCUITS

2 cups almond flour

2 teaspoons aluminum-free baking powder

$^1/_2$ teaspoon xanthan gum

1 teaspoon 1-for-1 allulose or monk fruit sweetener

1 teaspoon iodized sea salt

2 omega-3 eggs or vegan egg substitute

4 tablespoons ($^1/_2$ stick) butter or coconut oil, melted and cooled to lukewarm

2 tablespoons MCT oil

$^1/_4$ cup unsweetened goat's-milk yogurt or coconut yogurt

FOR THE GRAVY

$^1/_4$ cup olive oil

1 shallot, minced

1 pound mushrooms, diced (see Note)

1 teaspoon fresh thyme leaves

1 tablespoon minced fresh sage

1 tablespoon poultry seasoning

Iodized sea salt

1 (14-ounce) can unsweetened coconut cream

1 teaspoon Dijon mustard

1 teaspoon coconut aminos

Note: You can use cremini, white button, chanterelle, portobello, or trumpet mushrooms, or a combination.

1. Make the biscuits: Preheat the oven to 350°F. Line a baking sheet with parchment paper.
2. In a large bowl, combine the almond flour, baking powder, xanthan gum, sweetener, and salt.
3. In a separate bowl, whisk together the eggs, melted butter, MCT oil, and yogurt.
4. Add the wet ingredients to the dry ingredients and stir until a cohesive dough forms.
5. Using a cookie scoop, form the dough into 12 tablespoon-size balls, placing them on the prepared baking sheet as you go, keeping them several inches apart. Using your fingers, shape each ball into a biscuit shape.
6. Bake for 13 to 16 minutes, until golden brown and firm on top. Let cool until just warm before eating.
7. While the biscuits are baking, make the gravy: In a large skillet, heat the olive oil over medium-high heat. Add the shallot and mushrooms and cook, stirring occasionally, until the mushrooms are very brown and tender, 6 to 8 minutes.
8. Add the thyme, sage, poultry seasoning, and a pinch of salt and cook, stirring frequently, for 2 to 3 minutes, until the herbs are fragrant.
9. Add the coconut cream and reduce the heat to low. Cook for 3 to 5 minutes, until the sauce is thick and creamy, then stir in the mustard and coconut aminos.
10. Taste and add salt as needed before serving over the biscuits.

Broccoli Fritters with Avocado Dipping Sauce

This recipe uses riced broccoli to make deliciously savory fritters. You can rice the broccoli yourself or buy frozen broccoli rice—it's available in just about every grocery store these days. These fritters make a great snack or appetizer, and the sauce is addicting.

Serves 4

FOR THE FRITTERS

4 cups small broccoli florets, or $2^1/_2$ cups frozen broccoli rice

4 large omega-3 eggs, beaten

$^3/_4$ cup almond flour

2 tablespoons ground flaxseed

$^1/_2$ cup grated Manchego or goat's-milk cheddar cheese, or $^1/_4$ cup nutritional yeast (see Note)

2 teaspoons onion powder

1 teaspoon garlic powder

1 teaspoon iodized sea salt

$^1/_2$ teaspoon smoked paprika

$^1/_2$ teaspoon cracked black pepper

$^1/_4$ cup olive oil or coconut oil

FOR THE SAUCE

2 ripe avocados, pitted

Juice of 1 lemon

$^1/_4$ cup fresh parsley, finely chopped before measuring

$^1/_4$ cup fresh dill, finely chopped before measuring

1 tablespoon minced capers

2 tablespoons MCT oil

Dash of coconut aminos

Note: If you're using nutritional yeast in place of the cheese, add an additional tablespoon of ground flaxseed.

1. Make the fritters: Preheat the oven to 300°F.
2. In a food processor, pulse the broccoli until it is the consistency of rice (skip this step if you're using premade broccoli rice).
3. Transfer the broccoli rice to a large bowl, add the eggs, almond flour, flaxseed, cheese, and seasonings, and stir to combine.
4. Let the mixture rest for 5 to 10 minutes.
5. Meanwhile, make the sauce: With a potato masher or using a food processor, blend together the avocados and lemon juice until smooth and creamy. Fold in the parsley, dill, capers, MCT oil, and coconut aminos, cover, and set aside while you cook your fritters.
6. Heat half the oil in a large skillet over medium-high heat.
7. Spoon 2-tablespoon mounds of the broccoli mixture into the pan and carefully flatten them to make fritter or burger shapes. Do not crowd the pan; you'll use about half the mixture for this first round.
8. Cook the fritters for 3 to 4 minutes, then carefully flip and cook for 3 minutes more. Transfer to a baking sheet and pop into the oven to keep warm while you cook the remaining batter.
9. Serve the fritters immediately, with the dipping sauce.

Keto Crab Cakes

These crab cakes were inspired by the crab cake recipe in *The Plant Paradox Cookbook*—but with a keto-friendly twist. Make sure to give the mixture time to hydrate before shaping and chilling—and be prepared to use more coconut flour than the recipe calls for (it absorbs liquid a little differently, after all). I like to serve these with a side of Avocado Dipping Sauce (page 189) or a lightly dressed green salad.

Serves 2

12 ounces lump crabmeat, or 12 ounces hearts of palm (packed in brine, not sugar), drained and finely chopped
2 celery stalks, diced
$^1/_2$ yellow onion, diced (save 1 teaspoon for the sauce)
2 garlic cloves, crushed
2 teaspoons Old Bay seasoning
1 tablespoon ground flaxseed
2 tablespoons coconut flour, plus more if needed
1 tablespoon MCT oil
1 omega-3 or pasture-raised egg or vegan egg substitute
$^1/_4$ cup almond flour, plus more for coating
$^1/_4$ cup avocado oil

1. In a large bowl, stir together the crabmeat or hearts of palm, celery, onion, garlic, Old Bay, and flaxseed. Let stand for 5 minutes, then drain any liquid that has collected in the bowl.
2. Add the coconut flour, MCT oil, and egg and stir to incorporate. Let rest for 10 minutes, then form the mixture into cakes. It should easily hold together—if it's falling apart, add more coconut flour a teaspoon at a time until it comes together.

3. Form the crab or hearts of palm mixture into 8 evenly sized cakes. Gently pat almond flour onto the outside of each one, then refrigerate for 15 to 20 minutes.

4. Heat the avocado oil in a large skillet over medium-high heat. Cook the crab cakes until browned on the bottom, 3 to 4 minutes, then gently flip and cook on the second side for 3 to 4 minutes.

5. Reduce the heat to low and cook until a sharp knife inserted into the center of a crab cake comes out hot, 1 to 2 minutes more.

6. Serve hot.

Thai-Inspired Green Curry Shellfish Stew

Back when I ate takeout more often, one of my go-to dishes was Thai-inspired curry. I love the complex flavors in both red and green curries, and particularly love the way green curry tastes with wild-caught shellfish. Tahini gives this stew a really robust texture—perfect for a cool evening.

Serves 8

1 tablespoon sesame oil

1 red onion, thinly sliced

1 fennel bulb, thinly sliced

1 tablespoon minced fresh ginger

4 garlic cloves, pressed or minced

2 tablespoons Thai green curry paste

1 tablespoon tahini

8 ounces mussels, scrubbed and debearded

2 (14-ounce) cans unsweetened full-fat coconut milk

$^1/_2$ cup mushroom broth, chicken broth, or vegetable broth

6 ounces peeled wild-caught shrimp

8 ounces wild scallops in shells if you can get them (thawed frozen scallops are okay)

$1^1/_2$ cups packed thinly sliced collard greens

1 tablespoon fish sauce or coconut aminos

Small handful of basil or cilantro, chopped

Juice of 1 lime

$^1/_4$ cup MCT oil

1. Heat the sesame oil in a large soup pot over medium-high heat. Add the onion and fennel and cook until tender and translucent, 3 to 5 minutes. Add the ginger and garlic and cook until

translucent and fragrant, then add the curry paste and tahini and stir until well incorporated. Cook for 1 to 2 minutes, until very fragrant.

2. Add the mussels, coconut milk, and broth. Cover and cook for 6 to 10 minutes, until the mussels have opened.

3. Add the shrimp, scallops, collard greens, and fish sauce. Cover and cook for 4 to 6 minutes more, until the shrimp are cooked through and the collard greens are wilted.

4. Uncover and simmer for 3 to 4 minutes, until thickened slightly. Remove from the heat and discard any mussels that have not opened.

5. Add the basil and lime juice. Drizzle with the MCT oil and serve.

Mushroom and Goat Cheese Miracle Noodles

This is my riff on the popular pasta dish that's been sweeping TikTok and food blogs recently. By using roasted mushrooms instead of tomatoes, this dish takes on a meaty umami note that's perfect with shirataki noodles—and really satisfying to eat.

Serves 4

1 pound sliced brown button (cremini) mushrooms
$^1/_2$ cup extra-virgin olive oil
4 garlic cloves, minced
2 tablespoons fresh thyme leaves
1 (7-ounce) block feta cheese (see Note)
1 teaspoon iodized sea salt
1 teaspoon freshly ground black pepper
2 bags shirataki noodles of choice
$^1/_4$ cup coarsely chopped fresh basil, for serving

1. Preheat the oven to 400°F.
2. In a large baking dish, combine the mushrooms, $^1/_4$ cup of the olive oil, the garlic, and the thyme. Make space for the feta in the center of the mushrooms (not on top of them) and drizzle with the remaining $^1/_4$ cup oil. Sprinkle the mushrooms and feta with the salt and pepper.
3. Bake for 35 to 40 minutes, until the mushrooms are tender and crisp at the edges and the feta is very soft.
4. While mushrooms are cooking, bring a pot of salted water to a boil.
5. Rinse the noodles under cold running water for 2 to 3 minutes, then add them to the pot of boiling water and cook for 2 to 3

minutes. Drain and transfer to a dry pan. Cook over medium-low heat, stirring, to dry out the noodles.

6. Mash the feta with a fork and stir to combine with the mushrooms. Add a little hot water if it needs help loosening up (DO NOT add cold water if you're cooking in a glass dish, as this could cause the dish to shatter).

7. Toss the mushroom-feta mixture with the shirataki noodles and serve topped with the basil.

Note: To make this dish vegan: Omit the feta and roast the mushrooms as directed. While the mushrooms are cooking, bring 1 (14-ounce) can of unsweetened coconut cream to a simmer. Add $1/4$ cup nutritional yeast and $1/2$ teaspoon mustard powder. Toss the sauce with the mushroom mixture and noodles before serving.

Crispy Roasted Cabbage with Lemon-Herb Pesto

Not too long ago, I stumbled across a recipe for roasted cabbage on the Smitten Kitchen website. It was just about compliant with my plan, and I was excited to try it. This variation has become one of my weeknight go-tos. The addition of fresh herbs really balances out the salty roasted cabbage—and my favorite part is, you can use any herb in your fridge for the pesto.

Serves 4

1 head cabbage (any variety), cut into 8 to 10 wedges

3 tablespoons extra-virgin olive oil

1 teaspoon iodized sea salt, plus more to taste

$^1/_4$ cup MCT oil

Zest and juice of 1 lemon

1 garlic clove, minced

2 tablespoons grated Parmesan or Manchego cheese or nutritional
yeast

$^1/_4$ cup minced pistachios or toasted walnuts

3 tablespoons minced fresh parsley

1 tablespoon minced fresh basil or mint

1. Preheat the oven to 425°F.
2. On a baking sheet, toss the cabbage with 2 tablespoons of the olive oil and the salt. Spread into a single layer and bake for 8 to 10 minutes per side, turning once, until the cabbage is browned and crisp at the edges and tender all the way through.
3. While the cabbage is baking, in a small bowl, combine the remaining 1 tablespoon olive oil, the MCT oil, lemon zest,

lemon juice, and garlic until the garlic is evenly dispersed in the oil.

4. Fold in the cheese, nuts, and herbs to make a chunky "pesto." It should be thick, rustic, and spoonable, but not pourable.

5. Remove the cabbage from the oven. Spoon the pesto onto the cabbage before serving.

Pistachio-Crusted Goat Cheese Salad

There was a time when goat cheese "croutons" were a super-trendy salad topping—and you know what? They stand the test of time. In this new variation, the addition of orange zest really pops with the pistachio "breading" on the goat cheese.

Serves 4

1 (4-ounce) log fresh goat cheese
$^1/_2$ cup shelled pistachios
$^1/_4$ cup almond flour
$1^1/_2$ teaspoons psyllium husk powder
4 tablespoons olive oil
2 tablespoons MCT oil
Juice of 1 lemon
1 teaspoon Dijon mustard
2 tablespoons red wine vinegar
Zest of 1 orange
8 cups arugula
1 fennel bulb, shaved
1 avocado, diced
$^1/_4$ cup pomegranate seeds (optional, if in season)

1. Cut the goat cheese log crosswise into 8 equal-size coins. Set aside.
2. In a food processor or high-speed blender, pulse the pistachios until finely chopped (you can do this with a sharp knife, but it takes much longer).
3. Transfer the pistachios to a small bowl, add the almond flour and psyllium, and whisk to combine.

4. Coat each goat cheese coin with the nut mixture, then refrigerate for at least 20 minutes or up to overnight.

5. Meanwhile, in a jar with a tight-fitting lid, combine 2 tablespoons of the olive oil, the MCT oil, lemon juice, mustard, vinegar, and orange zest. Cover and shake to combine.

6. In a large bowl, combine the arugula, fennel, and avocado. Add the dressing and toss to coat. Set aside.

7. Heat the remaining 2 tablespoons of olive oil in a skillet over medium heat. Add the goat cheese and cook for 1 to 2 minutes per side, until the nuts are fragrant and toasty.

8. Top the salad with the goat cheese and pomegranate seeds (if using), then serve.

MCT-Infused Salad Dressings

Adding MCT oil to salad dressing is an easy way to boost your ketone production. For these dressings, I went beyond the classic vinaigrette (which I love) for two plays on restaurant favorites: a ginger-sesame dressing and a classic tangy ranch.

Ginger-Sesame Dressing

Serves 8

1 small bunch scallions
1 celery stalk
1 (2-inch) knob fresh ginger, peeled
1 tablespoon miso paste
2 tablespoons 1-for-1 allulose or monk fruit sweetener
2 tablespoons toasted or regular sesame oil
2 tablespoons MCT oil
$^{1}/_{4}$ cup rice vinegar
Coconut aminos

1. Combine all the ingredients except the coconut aminos in a high-speed blender or food processor and blend until smooth and creamy (this may take a couple of minutes, depending on your blender). If the dressing is too thick, add a bit of water to loosen it up.
2. Taste and add coconut aminos to increase the saltiness, if needed.
3. Serve or transfer to a jar and refrigerate for up to 1 week.

MCT Coconut Ranch

Serves 8

1 (14-ounce) can unsweetened coconut cream

2 tablespoons minced shallot

1 garlic clove, minced

Juice of $\frac{1}{2}$ lemon

2 tablespoons MCT oil

$1\frac{1}{2}$ teaspoons Dijon mustard

3 tablespoons chopped fresh chives

$1\frac{1}{2}$ tablespoons chopped fresh parsley

$1\frac{1}{2}$ tablespoons chopped fresh basil

1 tablespoon chopped fresh dill

1 teaspoon iodized sea salt

Freshly ground black pepper

1. In a deep bowl, whisk together the coconut cream, shallot, garlic, lemon juice, MCT oil, and mustard until well combined. Fold in the chives, parsley, basil, and dill. The mixture should be creamy but pourable. If it's too thick, add water a teaspoon at a time to thin it.
2. Add the salt and season with pepper.
3. Serve or transfer to a jar and refrigerate for up to 1 week.

Sauerkraut Casserole

Even if you don't count yourself among the many who love the tang-iness of sauerkraut, this casserole will change your mind! Creamy, cheesy, and satisfying, it comes together quickly and is absolutely craveable.

Serves 6

$^1/_4$ cup extra-virgin olive oil

8 ounces mushrooms (creminis, chanterelles, or portobellos work great), diced

1 yellow onion, diced

1 bay leaf

1 teaspoon mustard powder

$^1/_2$ teaspoon paprika

1 teaspoon freshly ground black pepper

$^1/_4$ teaspoon grated nutmeg

2 pounds sauerkraut, drained

2 (14-ounce) cans unsweetened coconut cream

$^1/_4$ cup grated pecorino or Parmesan cheese or nutritional yeast

4 omega-3 eggs or vegan egg substitute

1 cup walnuts, chopped

1. Preheat the oven to 375°F. Lightly grease a 2-quart gratin dish or brownie pan.
2. Heat the olive oil in a large pot over medium-high heat. Add the mushrooms, onion, and bay leaf and cook, stirring frequently, until the mushrooms are tender and the onion is translucent and fragrant, about 7 minutes.
3. Add the mustard powder, paprika, pepper, nutmeg, and sauer-

kraut and cook for 5 minutes more. Remove from the heat. Remove and discard the bay leaf.

4. Add the coconut cream and the cheese. Stir to combine, then stir in the eggs.

5. Transfer to the prepared dish and bake for about 35 minutes, or until the gratin is set and a little jiggly.

6. Sprinkle with the walnuts and bake until the walnuts are toasty and the top of the gratin is brown, 5 to 10 minutes more.

7. Serve and enjoy.

Coconut Curry with Lamb or Quorn

I love the spiciness (it's just right, not over the top) and versatility of this satisfying curry dish. For a vegan option, swap in Quorn for the lamb. And don't skip toasting the spices—it may seem minor, but it blooms the spices and opens up their fragrance and flavor.

Serves 4-6

3 to 4 teaspoons avocado oil

$^1/_3$ teaspoon mustard seeds

$^1/_3$ teaspoon cumin seeds

1 green cardamom pod

3 whole cloves

1 red onion, minced

3 garlic cloves, minced

1 pound ground lamb, or 1 bag Quorn crumbles

8 ounces mushrooms, minced

$^1/_2$ teaspoon ground turmeric

$^1/_3$ teaspoon ground cinnamon

1 teaspoon cracked black pepper

2 cups unsweetened full-fat coconut milk

2 cups baby spinach or shredded kale leaves

Iodized sea salt

1. Heat 1 teaspoon of the avocado oil in a large stainless-steel pan over low heat. Add the mustard seeds and cumin seeds and toast for about 20 seconds. Add the cardamom and cloves and toast, stirring frequently, for 1 minute. Remove from the heat. Pulse the spices in a spice grinder until finely ground.

2. Pour the remaining oil into the pan and add the onion and

garlic. Cook, stirring, over medium heat until the onion is golden brown, 2 to 4 minutes.

3. Add the lamb and mushrooms and cook for 7 to 8 minutes, until the lamb is browned and crisp at the edges. Add the ground spice mix, turmeric, cinnamon, and black pepper and stir.

4. Add the coconut milk and spinach. Cook for 15 to 20 minutes, until the mushrooms are tender.

5. Taste, season with salt, and serve.

Hemp Heart Tabbouleh

Hemp hearts are delicious and loaded with protein. This raw dish is based on the classic Middle Eastern salad and features the same tangy, fresh, herbal flavor, minus the lectin-heavy tomatoes and cucumbers. (I always make a double batch to guarantee leftovers!)

Serves 6

1 cup hulled hemp hearts
1 red onion, diced
2 celery stalks, diced
1 cup fresh mint, minced before measuring
1 cup fresh parsley, minced before measuring
$^1/_4$ cup scallions or fresh chives, minced before measuring
Juice of 1 lemon
1 teaspoon red wine vinegar
1 garlic clove, minced
2 tablespoons MCT oil
2 tablespoons extra-virgin olive oil
Sea salt and freshly ground black pepper

1. In a large bowl, toss together the hemp hearts, onion, celery, mint, parsley, and scallions. Set aside.
2. In a small bowl, whisk together the lemon juice, vinegar, garlic, MCT oil, and olive oil so the garlic is well distributed.
3. Pour the dressing over the hemp heart mixture and toss to combine. Taste and season with salt and pepper as needed.
4. Serve immediately or cover and refrigerate for a day to let the flavors meld and make it really special.

Pork Chops with Fennel and Red Wine Reduction

This simple, flavorful dish is an absolutely fantastic dinner party entrée—and it's simple enough to cook any night of the week. If you prefer not to cook with wine, consider using pasture-raised beef broth or mushroom broth and the juice of one lemon for a slightly different but equally delicious option.

Serves 4

4 bone-in pasture-raised pork chops, or 4 to 6 portobello
   mushroom caps
$^1/_2$ teaspoon iodized sea salt, plus more as needed
4 tablespoons olive oil
1 fennel bulb, thinly sliced
3 garlic cloves, minced
2 tablespoons minced fresh parsley (preferably flat-leaf)
Zest of 1 orange
$^1/_2$ teaspoon fennel seeds
1 cup dry red wine

1. Season both sides of the pork chops with the salt and set aside (skip this step if you're using portobellos).
2. Heat 2 tablespoons of the olive oil in a large saute pan over medium-high heat. Pat the pork chops dry, then sear until golden brown on each side, 2 to 3 minutes per side. Remove from the heat and set aside. (If using portobellos, sear until crisp on both sides, 2 to 3 minutes per side.)
3. Add the remaining 2 tablespoons olive oil to the pan, then add the sliced fennel and cook for 2 to 3 minutes, until it begins to wilt.

4. Add the garlic, parsley, orange zest, and fennel seeds and cook for 2 to 3 minutes, until the sliced fennel is tender and the mixture is very fragrant.

5. Return the pork chops (or mushrooms) to the pan, add $^3/_4$ cup of the wine, and reduce the heat to low. Simmer, turning the chops from time to time to ensure even cooking and coating with the red wine, until the wine has almost completely evaporated and the pork has reached 145°F at its thickest part (or until the mushrooms are tender). Remove the pork chops (or mushrooms) from the pan and set aside.

6. Add the remaining $^1/_4$ cup red wine and let it reduce until syrupy.

7. Pour the wine-fennel mixture over the pork or mushrooms and serve immediately.

Naan-Inspired Keto Flatbread

This flatbread recipe was inspired by two things: garlic naan and keto fathead doughs. The mozzarella gives the bread the stretchy, slightly chewy texture that makes it so delicious. For the vegan variation, be aware that the dough will be a little hard to handle, but don't worry—the finished product will be absolutely delicious.

Makes 8 flatbreads

$2^1/_2$ cups shredded mozzarella cheese (see Note)
$^1/_2$ cup shredded Manchego cheese
$^1/_4$ cup unsweetened full-fat coconut milk
$1^1/_2$ cups almond flour
1 tablespoon aluminum-free baking powder
2 large omega-3 eggs, at room temperature
2 tablespoons extra-virgin olive oil
2 garlic cloves, minced

Note: Make sure your mozzarella is from Italy, or was made using either buffalo or A2 cow's milk, or better yet, goat mozzarella, which is now sold everywhere.

1. Preheat the oven to 350°F. Line a large baking sheet with parchment paper or a silicone baking mat.
2. Combine the mozzarella, Manchego, and coconut milk in a small saucepan and heat over low heat, whisking continuously, until the cheeses have melted and the mixture is well combined, about 5 minutes. Transfer the cheese mixture to a large bowl and let cool for 2 to 3 minutes.
3. Add the almond flour, baking powder, and eggs to the cheese mixture and stir until a smooth, cohesive dough forms.

4. Divide the dough into 8 pieces and shape into balls. Flatten the balls into rounds and place them on the prepared baking sheet.

5. Bake for 16 to 18 minutes. While the flatbreads are baking, combine the garlic and olive oil.

6. When the flatbreads have puffed up and are almost golden brown, brush them with the olive oil mixture and bake for 2 minutes more.

7. Remove from the oven and let cool for 8 to 10 minutes before serving.

Vegan Variation

2 cups shredded vegan mozzarella (such as Kite Hill)

$^{1}/_{4}$ cup unsweetened full-fat coconut milk

$1^{1}/_{2}$ cups almond flour

2 tablespoons psyllium husk powder

$1^{1}/_{2}$ teaspoons xanthan gum

1 teaspoon aluminum-free baking powder

$^{1}/_{4}$ cup unsweetened coconut yogurt

2 tablespoons extra-virgin olive oil

2 garlic cloves, minced

1. Preheat the oven to 350°F. Line a large baking sheet with parchment paper or a silicone baking mat.

2. Combine the vegan cheese and coconut milk in a small saucepan and heat over low heat, whisking continuously, until the cheese has melted and the mixture is well combined, about 5 minutes. Transfer the cheese mixture to a large bowl and let cool for 2 to 3 minutes.

3. In a separate bowl, whisk together the almond flour, psyllium, xanthan gum, and baking powder. Add the yogurt and stir to combine (it won't incorporate fully yet, but do your best).

4. Add the cheese mixture and mix until a smooth, cohesive dough forms.

5. Divide the dough into 8 pieces and shape into balls. Flatten the balls into rounds and place them on the prepared baking sheet.

6. While the flatbreads are baking, combine the garlic and olive oil.

7. When the flatbreads have puffed up and are almost golden brown, brush them with the olive oil mixture and bake for 2 minutes more.

8. Remove from the oven and let cool for 8 to 10 minutes before serving.

Passion Fruit Coconut Ice Cream

This tasty nondairy frozen treat is perfect for those nights when you just *need* a little something sweet at the end of a long day. Because it doesn't contain sugar, this "ice cream" freezes a little hard, so make sure to leave it out at room temperature for a bit before scooping—or enjoy it straight from the ice cream machine for the best possible texture.

Serves 8

1 (13.5-ounce) can unsweetened full-fat coconut milk

2 tablespoons macadamia nut butter or tahini

$^1/_2$ cup 1-for-1 allulose or monk fruit sweetener

$^1/_4$ teaspoon iodized sea salt, plus more as needed

$^1/_4$ teaspoon xanthan gum

1 (13.5-ounce) can unsweetened coconut cream, refrigerated overnight

$^1/_4$ cup unsweetened shredded coconut, toasted (optional)

1 tablespoon pure vanilla extract

1 tablespoon barrel-aged rum

1 cup passion fruit puree with seeds (from about 6 ripe passion fruit; see Note)

Note: If you can't find fresh passion fruit, swap in frozen unsweetened passion fruit puree.

1. Place a metal bowl in the fridge or freezer. If using an ice cream machine, make sure your core is frozen through.
2. In a high-speed blender, combine the coconut milk, nut butter, and sweetener and blend until well combined.
3. Transfer to a saucepan and heat over low heat until barely

simmering. While whisking continuously, add the salt and xanthan gum and whisk until fully combined and dissolved. If the mixture is lumpy, transfer it back to the blender and blend until smooth.

4. Cover and let cool completely. The mixture will thicken to a jellylike consistency. Don't worry—your ice cream will NOT feel like that.

5. Open the can of chilled coconut cream and pour off any coconut water. Spoon the thick white coconut cream into the chilled bowl and whip the cream until soft peaks form.

6. Gently fold in the shredded coconut, vanilla, rum, a tiny pinch of salt, and the cooled coconut–nut butter mixture.

7. **If using an ice cream machine:** Transfer the mixture to the machine and freeze according to the manufacturer's instructions—it should take about 15 minutes. When the ice cream is almost set, add the passion fruit and let the paddle fold it in. Serve immediately for a soft-serve consistency or transfer to an airtight container and freeze for 20 minutes, or until scoopable.

8. **To freeze without an ice cream machine:** Transfer the mixture to a freezer-safe container and fold in the passion fruit to create ribbons. Freeze for at least 4 hours, stirring every 20 minutes or so, until frozen. Let sit at room temperature for 12 minutes before serving.

MCT Brownies with Spiced Walnuts

I know it's super tempting to eat brownies hot out of the oven—but these are pretty delicate until they cool down, so resist the temptation! It's completely fine to make these without the candied nuts, but they're extra delicious with them.

Makes 16 brownies

FOR THE CANDIED NUTS

$^1/_2$ cup chopped walnuts

1 tablespoon omega-3 egg white or liquid from pressure-cooked beans (aquafaba)

2 tablespoons 1-for-1 allulose or monk fruit sweetener

$^1/_2$ teaspoon ground cinnamon

$^1/_2$ teaspoon iodized sea salt

$^1/_4$ teaspoon freshly ground black pepper

FOR THE BROWNIES

1 cup almond flour

$^1/_4$ cup plus 2 tablespoons unsweetened natural (non-Dutched) cocoa powder

1 teaspoon aluminum-free baking powder

$^1/_2$ teaspoon iodized sea salt

$^1/_3$ cup coconut oil or goat butter, melted

3 tablespoons MCT oil

$^2/_3$ cup 1-for-1 allulose or monk fruit sweetener

2 omega-3 eggs or vegan egg substitute

1 teaspoon pure vanilla extract

1. Make the candied nuts: Preheat the oven to 350°F. Line a baking sheet with parchment paper or a silicone baking mat.

2. In a large bowl, combine the walnuts, egg white, sweetener, cinnamon, salt, and pepper and stir until the nuts are evenly coated with the spice mixture.

3. Spread the nuts evenly over the prepared baking sheet and bake, stirring occasionally, until fragrant but not burnt, 10 to 15 minutes. Remove from the oven and let cool; keep the oven on.

4. Make the brownies: Line an 8-inch square baking dish with parchment paper.

5. In a large bowl, whisk together the almond flour, cocoa powder, baking powder, and salt. Set aside.

6. In a saucepan, whisk together the coconut oil, MCT oil, and sweetener. Cook over low heat, stirring continuously, until the sweetener is incorporated into the oil and the mixture is no longer grainy. Remove from the heat.

7. Stir the oil mixture into the dry ingredients. Let rest until *just* warm.

8. Stir in the eggs, one at a time, then fold in the vanilla and spiced nuts.

9. Transfer to the prepared baking dish and bake for 20 to 25 minutes, until the center is firm and begins to crack and a toothpick inserted into the center comes out clean.

10. Let cool completely before slicing and serving.

Cinnamon Spice Mug Cake

The microwave mug cakes I've shared in my previous books quickly became reader favorites, so I've come up with another crowd-pleaser: cinnamon spice cake. This tasty cake combines the flavors of a classic coffee cake with a gooey, cinnamon roll–inspired frosting. I dare you not to try it!

Makes 1 mug cake

FOR THE CAKE:

1 tablespoon MCT oil

1 large omega-3 egg or Vegg egg replacer

$1/2$ teaspoon pure vanilla extract

3 tablespoons almond flour

1 tablespoon 1-for-1 allulose or monk fruit sweetener

$1/2$ teaspoon aluminum-free baking powder

$1/4$ teaspoon ground cinnamon

$1/4$ teaspoon ground ginger

$1/8$ teaspoon ground cloves

$1/8$ teaspoon iodized sea salt

FOR THE FROSTING

$1^1/2$ tablespoons tahini

$1/2$ teaspoon MCT oil (plain or vanilla flavored)

1 teaspoon powdered Swerve or 1-for-1 allulose or monk fruit
    sweetener, plus more if needed

$1/4$ teaspoon ground cinnamon, plus more if needed

1. Make the cake: In a microwave-safe mug, thoroughly combine the MCT oil, egg, vanilla, almond flour, sweetener, baking powder, cinnamon, ginger, cloves, and salt to form a smooth batter,

carefully scraping the sides and bottom of the mug to make sure all the flour is incorporated.

2. Make the frosting: Whisk together the tahini, MCT oil, sweetener, and cinnamon in a small bowl until well combined. Taste and add additional sweetener or cinnamon to your preference.

3. Microwave the cake for 80 to 90 seconds, watching carefully to make sure it rises but doesn't burn.

4. Drizzle with the frosting and enjoy.

Blueberry Soft-Serve

Back when I was trying to lose weight, I let myself indulge in a homemade "frozen" dessert made from frozen wild blueberries, cold nondairy milk, and a scoop of protein powder almost every night. This recipe is an improvement on that one, harnessing the power of MCTs in goat and sheep milk to make a delectable frozen dessert.

Serves 1 or 2

1 scoop unsweetened hemp protein powder (about 3 tablespoons)

$^1/_2$ cup unsweetened plain or vanilla goat, sheep, coconut, or Lavva yogurt

$^1/_2$ cup chilled unsweetened plain or vanilla coconut milk, Lavva milk, or almond-coconut milk

$^1/_2$ to 1 cup frozen organic wild blueberries

Allulose or Just Like Sugar

Combine the protein powder, yogurt, milk, and blueberries in a blender and blend to the consistency of soft-serve frozen yogurt (or mix in a bowl). Taste and add sweetener as desired, then enjoy immediately.

ACKNOWLEDGMENTS

Very much like its predecessor, *Unlocking the Keto Code*, as a book, wasn't supposed to happen. But the revelations of how ketones worked—not like a super fuel but as super signaling agents to tell mitochondria to uncouple, which I discovered while writing *The Energy Paradox*—mandated that I write this book and get it in your hands as quickly as possible. I initially received some help from my old collaborator Olivia Buehl, then I took it from there. But communicating just how important "uncoupling" mitochondria is to the lay reader (a difficult concept indeed!) needed the skills of Kayt Sukel, wordsmith extraordinaire, to hone and whittle my verbiage down to the hopefully easy-to-grasp pages you have just read. Thank you, both.

The recipes were once again contributed by working with Kathryn "Kate" Holzhauer, my head chef at GundryMD, this time with some fun ways to get more gut-buddy and uncoupling foods into you. Who knew how delicious uncoupling could taste? A win-win-win for your taste buds, your microbiome, and your mitochondria. Thanks again, Kate!

The team at Harper Wave keeps going and going, bringing this home during the COVID-19 pandemic. Of course, thanks again to my publisher, Karen Rinaldi; vice president of marketing Brian Perrin; publicity director Yelena Nesbit; art director Milan Bozic, who has designed all the Paradox covers; editorial assistant Emma Kupor; and, of course, vice president and editorial director Julie Will, who has been at the helm for all seven of my bestsellers. It's a great team to have behind me and supporting me, even more so this time, when we decided as a group that this book needed to stand apart from the Paradox series, as its content needed a new look and feel.

The team at the International Heart and Lung Institute and the Center for Restorative Medicine in Palm Springs and Santa Barbara, California, continued to step up to bat big-time with COVID-19 still knocking on our doors. Led by my longtime executive assistant Susan Lokken and my now longtime colleague and physician's assistant Mitsu Killian-Jacobo, our team of Tanya Marta; Cindy Crosby; my daughter, Melissa Perko; Jessenia Parra; Nellie Melero; and Natalie Garcia kept the doors open, safe, and welcoming all this time. Thank you again, from the bottom of my and, I'm sure, our patients' hearts. And to the "blood suckers," Laurie Acuna, Lynn Visk, and Samantha Acuna, who kept the blood tests flowing, despite risks.

Thanks also to my accountant and CFO, Joe Tames, and my attorney and friend, Dave Baron, who keep the doors open.

All my work is guided by my longtime agent and early believer, Shannon Marven, president of Dupree Miller, who believed, once again, that this book needed to be written. And thank you to her great assistant and coworker Rebecca Silensky, who gets things done! Thanks again, and I can't wait for the "next one"!

Finally, I cannot express enough thanks to the six-hundred-plus people at GundryMD who have made me, GundryMD.com, and *The Dr. Gundry Podcast* the trusted sources for health and supplement advice for hundreds of millions of people daily. Despite the pandemic, a few of us arrive, screened and ready, every Friday at GundryMD, to bring you up-to-date information so vital to your health, especially now. And while I can't mention all of you here, thank you for continuing to service and support the millions of GundryMD family with our products and knowledge during this time. A heartfelt thanks to my right-hand woman at GundryMD, Lanee Lee Neil, who protects and manages me along with Kate mentioned above, and my great team of writers who keep the information flowing. And a well-deserved shout-out to Rebecca Reinbold and her team at Stanton and Co, who are always getting the press's attention about my latest mind-bending findings.

As I've said in all my Paradox books and now in *Unlocking the Keto Code*, nothing you read on any of these pages would be possible without my patients and readers letting me learn from them over the last twenty-plus years of practicing restorative medicine, which I continue to do full time, six days a week (yes, even Saturdays and Sundays). Thank you all again.

Finally, I wouldn't be able to do any of this without the love and support of my soul mate and wife, Penny. How she tolerates all this is astonishing! Shockingly, the minute *The Energy Paradox* was wrapped up, *Unlocking the Keto Code* writing began. Penny, your patience is appreciated! That's a lot of hours locked up in my office, before and after patients.

And for those of you who follow such things, the "pack" is back to the usual four dogs, following the death, at age nineteen, of our first rescue, George II, replaced by our new rescue, a toy poodle, Okie Dokie. And if you see us out on the streets of Palm Springs or Montecito, yes, my real profession is dog walker!

And, for those of you who actually read this far, Pearl, our huge old female Labradoodle, is the latest beneficiary of uncoupling, which reversed a "normally" life-ending bladder cancer discovered a year ago when she couldn't empty her bladder. No surgery, no chemo, no keto diet, just uncoupling supplements and she's "peeing like a racehorse." No wonder I had to write this book—Pearl made me!

SUPPLEMENTS

While the best way to harness mitochondrial uncoupling is through eating the polyphenol-rich, polyamine-containing, and fermented foods we discussed in chapter 9, you may find it helpful to add some supplements to your arsenal as you work to unlock the keto code. Just note that supplementation can be helpful, but is not necessary, and if you do choose to add some supplements to your diet, be sure to seek out reputable, high-quality products with known ingredients.

YOUR KETO CODE PROGRAM SUPPLEMENTS

Vitamin D$_3$

Most patients who visit me are deficient in vitamin D—heck, the majority of Americans are! And all my autoimmune and metabolically inflexible patients show low vitamin D levels. Low vitamin D is strongly correlated with metabolic syndrome, as well as susceptibility to infection (including the novel coronavirus COVID-19).[1] That's why I recommend that everyone aim for a vitamin D level of 100 to 150 ng/ml. Regular exposure to sunlight is one easy and free way to increase vitamin D production in the body—and you can also enjoy foods like mushrooms, which are abundant in this nutrient. Unfortunately, both are insufficient to get you to the levels you need.

To supplement your vitamin D intake, I recommend a bare minimum of 5,000 IU (125 mcg) of vitamin D_3. For my patients with leaky gut, I actually start them at 10,000 IU (250 mcg).[2] Even at that high a dosage, I have yet to see vitamin D toxicity—even at levels greater than 200 ng/ml.

Given that vitamin D uncouples mitochondria, this should definitely be something to add to your daily regimen. It works even better when combined with vitamin K_2!

Vitamin K_2

This vitamin not only helps your body make the most of calcium but is also an essential cofactor in mitochondrial function—and, of course, an uncoupler in its own right. This vitamin is largely missing from the modern Westernized diet. You can find it in grass-fed milk products, including butter and cheeses, but it is easy to get the levels you need by taking a K_2 supplement. A daily dose of 100 mcg of both the MK4 and MK7 varieties should suffice—but don't hesitate to take larger doses if you want.

Long-Chain Omega-3s

Most people are profoundly deficient in omega-3 fatty acids like eicosapentaenoic acid (EPA) and, even more important, docosahexaenoic acid (DHA) and docosapentaenoic acid (DPA). Given that the human brain is about 60 percent fat—half of which is DHA—the lack of these nutrients is a grave problem. Studies show that people with the highest levels of omega-3 fats in their blood have bigger brains, better memories, and improved cognitive function over those with the lowest levels. Why? Because the mitochondria in their neurons are being actively uncoupled by these vital fats.

It's also important to get arachidonic acid (AA). Many people refer to this long-chain omega-3 as a "bad fat." I assure you, this reputation is quite unfounded. AA makes up an equally significant portion of the fat in your brain and also works as an uncoupler. Egg yolks and shellfish are great sources of this particular fat.

I recommend supplementing with a fish oil that is molecularly distilled. Brands like Nature's Bounty, OmegaVia, and Carlson offer this kind of supplement. For vegans, there are also good algae-derived DHA, EPA, and DPA capsules.

Whether you choose a fish-based or algae-based supplement, aim for at least 1,000 mg of DHA per day—and if you want, throw in another 1,000 mg of EPA. And as I mentioned earlier, arachidonic acid supplementation has been linked to improved cognition in elderly men, so I would also suggest considering a 250 mg dose of AA each day.

Ketone salts

Premade ketones are a great way to help boost ketone levels, especially early in the program when your own ketone production may not be up to speed. Ketones can be supplemented in the form of salts or esters, but I don't recommend the esters because, frankly, they taste awful and are quite expensive. Ketone salts, however, are readily available as powders and capsules. Consider a dose of about 10,000 mg mixed ketone salts (BHB) in the morning when starting the Keto Code program. Think of it as a way of kick-starting ketone production, increasing the levels circulating in your system until your body is in a position to start producing its own.

Coenzyme Q10 (CoQ10), Ubiquinol, or Pyrroloquinoline quinone (PQQ)

These are supplementary forms of a coenzyme important in making energy; recent evidence shows that CoQ10 is also an essential factor in activating multiple mitochondrial uncoupling proteins. In general, 100 to 300 mg of CoQ10, 100 mg of ubiquinol, or 20 mg of PQQ is an ample dose to provide strong mitochondrial support.[3] If you are taking a statin drug, you are likely depleted in this coenzyme. Ask your doctor to measure it in your blood work; if your levels are low, you may need to increase your supplement dose to 300 mg.

Liver protectors

A large proportion of my first-time patients suffer from nonalcoholic steatohepatitis (NASH) or nonalcoholic fatty liver disease (NAFLD). This problem is usually caused by a combination of mitochondrial overload, high fructose/sugar consumption, and leaky gut. If you have elevated liver enzymes or have had an ultrasound that shows fatty liver, there is a war being waged in your liver cells—and the main casualties are your mitochondria. To combat this, I recommend the polyphenol milk thistle and a component of orange peel called D-limonene—both at a dose of about 1,000 mg a day. They are remarkably effective at reducing hepatic inflammation by uncoupling mitochondria. Other uncouplers for the liver mitochondria include artichoke extract and dandelion extract.

Berberine and Quercetin

Berberine, a compound found in bayberry and Oregon grape root (not to be confused with grape seed extract, another great polyphenol mitochondrial uncoupler), and quercetin, found in foods like onions, apples, and the pith of citrus fruits, are both major drivers of mitochondrial repair and mitogenesis. The recommended dose for either is 500 mg twice a day. (By the way, for you allergy sufferers, quercetin is one of the best nonsedating natural antihistamines around. You should give it a try!)

Polyphenols

Where to start? I recommend grape seed extract, maritime pine bark extract (sometimes marketed by the brand name Pycnogenol), and resveratrol, the polyphenol found in red wine. You can find these supplements at stores like Costco, Trader Joe's, and Whole Foods, and on many online sites. I recommend taking 100 mg per day of both grape seed extract and resveratrol, and between 25 to 100 mg per day of pine bark extract.

In my opinion, the best resveratrol product on the market is Longevinex—which I have personally taken for at least fifteen years. I have no relationship with the company, but I am impressed by the research of its owner, Bill Sardi. As you may recall, resveratrol, as well as other small molecules in red wine like quercetin, activate sirtuin genes like SIRT1, which slow the process of aging in cells, by uncoupling mitochondria.

Other great polyphenol additions are green tea extract, cocoa powder, cinnamon, mulberry, and pomegranate.

Other Supplements to Consider

There are a lot of supplements out there, many of which promise good health and long life. Not all of them are mitochondrial uncouplers, however. As part of the Keto Code program, I recommend these uncoupling supplements, all of which I personally take.

7-HMR lignans (from Norwegian spruce)

81 mg enteric-coated aspirin

Aged garlic extract

Agmatine

Akkermansia capsules, Pendulum Health

Allithiamine (a form of vitamin B_1)

Alpha-carotene

Alpha-GPC

Amla (contained in GundryMD Active Heart)

Apigenin

Artichoke extract

Ashwagandha

Benfotiamine (a form of vitamin B_1)

Black cumin seed oil

Black raspberry

Brown seaweed

Butyric acid (as contained in GundryMD BioComplete 3)

Camu camu

Carbon 60 (myVitalC)

Cardamom

Celery seed capsules

Cloves

Coffee fruit extract

Cranberry seed oil

Fatty15 (C15)

Fenugreek and thyme

Fisetin

Fucoidan

Gingko biloba

Ginseng

Glucomannan (a prebiotic fiber)

GundryMD Active Advantage (CoQ10, mixed D-tocopherols and tocotrienols [vitamin E] and astaxanthin)

GundryMD Advanced Basil Formula

GundryMD Advanced Circulation Formula (L-citrulline, beet root powder, hawthorn berry, horny goat weed—you can laugh now, if you actually read this—pomegranate, Korean ginseng, cayenne)

GundryMD Citrus Polyphenols

GundryMD Complete Liver Support (milk thistle, L-limonene, dandelion root extract)

GundryMD Energy Renew (as D-ribose, N-acetyl-carnitine, BettaBerries antioxidant blend)

GundryMD Heart Defense (cocoa, flaxseed, coffee fruit extract, inulin)

GundryMD Herbal Mood Support (L-theanine, bacopa, rhodiola)

GundryMD M-Vitality mushroom blend

GundryMD MCT Wellness

GundryMD MCT creamer or other MCT creamer

GundryMD Metabolic Advanced (cinnamon bark, berberine, turmeric, chromium, selenium, zinc)

GundryMD Mito X (NAC, gynostemma, shilajit, L-glutathione, pau d'arco, PQQ, NADH)

GundryMD Peak Mobility Plus (hop extract, boswellia [Indian frankincense])

GundryMD Red Superfruit Polyphenols

Hops extract (included as part of GundryMD Peak Mobility Plus)

Jarrow Formulas N-A-C Sustain (may be temporarily hard to find because of the FDA)

L-glutathione

Low-dose Lithium

Lutein

Luteolin complex with rutin

Melatonin

Mitopure (urolithin-A)

Moringa

Mulberry extract

Mushrooms: coriolus (turkey tail), lion's mane, chaga, reishi

Myrosinase-activated SGS (broccoli seed extract)

Naringin

Nutmeg

Oil of oregano

Omega-7 (sea buckthorn oil)

Parsley capsules

Pomegranate seed oil

Potassium magnesium aspartate

PQQ

Pterostilbene

Quercetin

R-alpha-lipoic acid

Relora (magnolia bark extract and *Phellodendron amurense*)

Retinol-A (a form of vitamin A)

Rosemary extract

Saffron extract

Sage leaf extract

Sesame seed lignans

Silk protein complex

Spermadine

Triphala

NOTES

CHAPTER 2: KETONES ARE NOT A SUPER FUEL

1. Theodore B. VanItallie and Thomas H. Nufert, "Ketones: Metabolism's Ugly Duckling," *Nutrition Reviews* 61, no. 10 (2003): 327–41.
2. Kevin Loria, "The True Story of a Man Who Survived Without Any Food For 382 Days," *Business Insider*, March 2, 2017, https://www.sciencealert.com/the-true-story-of-a-man-who-survived-without-any-food-for-382-days.
3. Oliver E. Owen, "Ketone Bodies as a Fuel for the Brain During Starvation," *Biochemistry and Molecular Biology Education* 33, no. 4 (July 2005): 246–51, https://iubmb.onlinelibrary.wiley.com/doi/full/10.1002/bmb.2005.49403304246.
4. O. E. Owen and George A. Reichard Jr., "Human Forearm Metabolism During Progressive Starvation," *Journal of Clinical Investigation* 50, no. 7 (July 1971): 1536–1545, https://www.jci.org/articles/view/106639.
5. Ole Snorgaard et al., "Systematic Review and Meta-Analysis of Dietary Carbohydrate Restriction in Patients with Type 2 Diabetes," *BMJ Open Diabetes Research & Care* 5 (2017), https://drc.bmj.com/content/bmjdrc/5/1/e000354.full.pdf.
6. David Raubenheimer and Stephen J. Simpson, *Eat Like the Animals* (New York: Houghton Mifflin Harcourt, 2020).
7. Ibid.
8. Ole Snorgaard et al., "Systematic Review and Meta-Analysis of Dietary Carbohydrate Restriction in Patients with Type 2 Diabetes."
9. Michael Rosenbaum et al., "Glucose and Lipid Homeostasis and Inflammation in Humans Following an Isocaloric Ketogenic Diet," *Obesity* 27, no.

6 (June 2019): 971–81, https://www.ncbi.nlm.nih.gov/pmc/articles/PMC 6922028.

10. Lee Crosby et al., "Ketogenic Diets and Chronic Disease: Weighing the Benefits Against the Risks," *Frontiers in Nutrition* 8 (July 16, 2021): 702 802, https://doi.org/10.3389/fnut.2021.702802.

CHAPTER 3: HARNESSING OUR CELLS' PETITE POWERHOUSES

1. Joseph Pizzorno, "Mitochondria—Fundamental to Life and Health," *Integrative Medicine* 13, no. 2 (2014): 8–15.

2. Peter Rich, "Chemiosmotic Coupling: The Cost of Living," *Nature* 421 (2003): 583, https://www.nature.com/articles/421583a.

3. David G. Nicholls and Eduardo Rial, "A History of the First Uncoupling Protein, UCP1," *Journal of Bioenergetics and Biomembranes* 31 (1999): 399–406.

4. Martin D. Brand, "Uncoupling to Survive? The Role of Mitochondrial Inefficiency in Aging," *Experimental Gerontology* 35, no. 6–7 (2000): 811–820.

CHAPTER 4: THE POWER OF UNCOUPLING

1. Véronique Ouelletet et al., "Brown Adipose Tissue Oxidative Metabolism Contributes to Energy Expenditure During Acute Cold Exposure in Humans," *Journal of Clinical Investigation* 122, no. 2 (February 2012): 545–52, https://www.jci.org/articles/view/60433; Barbara Cannon and Jan Nedergaard, "Yes, Even Human Brown Fat Is on Fire!," *Journal of Clinical Investigation* 122, no. 2 (2012): 486–89, https://www.jci.org/articles/view/60941/pdf; Takeshi Yoneshiro et al., "BCAA Catabolism in Brown Fat Controls Energy Homeostasis Through SLC25A44," *Nature* 572 (2019): 614–19, https://www.nature.com/articles/s41586-019-1503-x.

2. Borut Poljsak, Dušan Šuput, and Irina Milisav, "Achieving the Balance Between ROS and Antioxidants: When to Use the Synthetic Antioxidants," *Oxidative Medicine and Cellular Longevity* (2013).

3. Zachary Pickell et al., "Histone Deacetylase Inhibitors: A Novel Strategy for Neuroprotection and Cardioprotection Following Ischemia/Reperfusion Injury," *Journal of the American Heart Association* 2020, no. 9 (May 2020): e016349, https://www.ahajournals.org/doi/10.1161/JAHA.120.016349.

4. W. C. Cutting, H. G. Mehrtens, and M. L. Tainter, "Actions and Uses of Dinitrophenol Promising Metabolic Applications," *JAMA* 101, no. 3

(July 15, 1933): 193–95, https://jamanetwork.com/journals/jama/article -abstract/244026.

5. Johann Grundlingh et al., "2,4-Dinitrophenol (DNP): A Weight Loss Agent with Significant Acute Toxicity and Risk of Death," *Journal of Medical Toxicology* 7, no. 3 (2011): 205–12, https://www.ncbi.nlm.nih.gov /pmc/articles/PMC3550200/.

6. Catherine E. Amara et al., "Mild Mitochondrial Uncoupling Impacts Cellular Aging in Human Muscles in Vivo," *Proceedings of the National Academy of Sciences* 104 , no. 3 (January 2007): 1057–62, https://www.pnas.org /content/104/3/1057.

7. Reiko Nakao et al., "Ketogenic Diet Induces Skeletal Muscle Atrophy via Reducing Muscle Protein Synthesis and Possibly Activating Proteolysis in Mice," *PNAS Science Reports* 9, no. 19652 (2019), https://doi.org/10.1038 /s41598-019-56166-8.

8. The Sinclair Lab Blavatnik Institute Genetics at Harvard Medical School, https://sinclair.hms.harvard.edu.

9. Jiejie Hao et al., "Hydroxytyrosol Promotes Mitochondrial Biogenesis and Mitochondrial Function in 3T3-L1 Adipocytes," *Journal of Nutritional Biochemistry* 21 (2009): 634-44, https://pubmed.ncbi.nlm.nih.gov/19576748/; Han Wern Lim, Hwee Ying Lim, Kim Ping Wong, "Uncoupling of Oxidative Phosphorylation by Curcumin: Implication of Its Cellular Mechanism of Action," *Biochemical and Biophysical Research Communications* 389, no. 1 (November 6, 2009): 187–92, https://pubmed.ncbi.nlm.nih.gov/19715674/; Lara Gibellini et al., "Natural Compounds Modulating Mitochondrial Functions," *Evidence-Based Complementary and Alternative Medicine* 2015 (2015), Article ID 527209, https://www.hindawi.com/journals/ecam/2015/527209/; Vidmantas Bendokas et al., "Anthocyanins: From Plant Pigments to Health Benefits at Mitochondrial Level," *Critical Reviews in Food Science and Nutrition* 60, no. 19 (2019): 3352–65, DOI: 10.1080/10408398.2019.1687421.

10. Ildefonso Guerrero-Encinas et al., "Protective Effects of Lacticaseibacillus casei CRL 431 Postbiotics on Mitochondrial Function and Oxidative Stress in Rats with Aflatoxin B1-Induced Oxidative Stress," *Probiotics and Antimicrobial Proteins* 13, no. 4, (August 2021).

11. Susanne Klaus and Mario Ost, "Mitochondrial Uncoupling and Longevity—A Role for Mitokines?," *Experimental Gerontology* 130 (February 2020), DOI: 10.1016/j.exger.2019.11079; Giuseppina Rose et al., "Further Support to the Uncoupling-to-Survive Theory: The Genetic Variation of Human UCP Genes Is Associated with Longevity," *PloS One* 6, no. 12 (2011): e29650, https://www.ncbi.nlm.nih.gov/pmc/articles/PMC 3246500/.

CHAPTER 5: THE KEYS THAT UNLOCK THE KETO CODE

1. Julie A. Mattison et al., "Impact of Caloric Restriction on Health and Survival in Rhesus Monkeys from the NIA Study," *Nature* 489, no. 7415 (2012): 318–21, https://www.ncbi.nlm.nih.gov/pmc/articles/PMC38329 85/.

2. Ricki J. Colman et al., "Caloric Restriction Delays Disease Onset and Mortality in Rhesus Monkeys," *Science* 325, no. 5937 (July 10, 2009): 201–204, https://science.sciencemag.org/content/325/5937/201.

3. Sarah J. Mitchell et al., "Daily Fasting Improves Health and Survival in Male Mice Independent of Diet Composition and Calories," *Cell Metabolism* 29, no. 1 (2019): 221–8.e3, https://pubmed.ncbi.nlm.nih.gov /30197301/.

4. Tatiana Moro et al., "Effects of Eight Weeks of Time-Restricted Feeding (16/8) on Basal Metabolism, Maximal Strength, Body Composition, Inflammation, and Cardiovascular Risk Factors in Resistance-Trained Males," *Journal of Translational Medicine* 14, no. 290 (2016), https://doi .org/10.1186/s12967-016-1044-0.

5. George J. Cahill Jr., "Fuel Metabolism in Starvation," *Annual Review of Nutrition* 26 (May 9, 2006): 1–22, https://thehealthsciencesacademy.org /wp-content/uploads/2015/07/Fuel-Metabolism-in-Starvation_Review ArticleTIMM2008-9Lazar-1.pdf.

6. Gemma Chiva-Blanch et al., "Effects of Wine, Alcohol and Polyphenols on Cardiovascular Disease Risk Factors: Evidences from Human Studies," *Alcohol and Alcoholism* 48, no. 3 (May/June 2013): 270–77, https://doi .org/10.1093/alcalc/agt007.

7. Yoona Kim, Jennifer B. Keogh, Peter M. Clifton, "Polyphenols and Glycemic Control," *Nutrients* 8, no. 1 (2016): 17, https://www.ncbi.nlm.nih.gov /pmc/articles/PMC4728631/.

8. David Vauzour, "Dietary Polyphenols as Modulators of Brain Functions: Biological Actions and Molecular Mechanisms Underpinning Their Beneficial Effects," *Oxidative Medicine and Cellular Longevity* 2012 (2012), DOI: 10.1155/2012/914273; N Hasima and B Ozpolat, "Regulation of Autophagy by Polyphenolic Compounds as a Potential Therapeutic Strategy for Cancer," *Cell Death & Disease* 5, no. 11 (November 6, 2014): e1509, https://www.ncbi.nlm.nih.gov/pmc/articles/PMC4260725/.

9. Johann Grundlingh et al., "2,4-Dinitrophenol (DNP): A Weight Loss Agent with Significant Acute Toxicity and Risk of Death," *Journal of Medical Toxicology* 7, no. 3 (2011): 205–12, https://www.ncbi.nlm.nih.gov /pmc/articles/PMC3550200.

10. Donald E. Moreland and William P. Novitzky, "Effects of Phenolic Acids,

Coumarins, and Flavonoids on Isolated Chloroplasts and Mitochondria," *Allelochemicals: Role in Agriculture and Forestry*, Chapter 23: 247–61, January 8, 1987. ACS *Symposium Series*, Vol. 330. ISBN13: 9780841209923. © 1987 American Chemical Society, https://pubs.acs.org/doi/10.1021/bk -1987-0330.ch023.

11. AWC Man, Y Zhou, N Xia, and H Li, "Involvement of Gut Microbiota, Microbial Metabolites and Interaction with Polyphenol Immunometabolism," *Nutrients* 12, no. 10 (2020): 3054, DOI: 10.3390/nu12103054.

12. Jiejie Hao et al., "Hydroxytyrosol Promotes Mitochondrial Biogenesis and Mitochondrial Function in 3T3-L1 Adipocytes," *Journal of Nutritional Biochemistry* 21, no. 7 (July 2010): 634–44, DOI: 10.1016/j.jnutbio .2009.03.012.

13. Ksenija Velickovic et al., "Caffeine Exposure Induces Browning Features in Adipose Tissue in Vitro and in Vivo," *Scientific Reports* 9, no. 9104 (2019), https://doi.org/10.1038/s41598-019-45540-1.

14. Lara Gibellini et al., "Natural Compounds Modulating Mitochondrial Functions," *Evidence-Based Complementary and Alternative Medicine* 2015 (2015), DOI: 10.1155/2015/527209.

15. Shan Wang et al., "Curcumin Promotes Browning of White Adipose Tissue in a Norepinephrine-Dependent Way," *Biochemical and Biophysical Research Communications* (2015): 1–7, http://kurmin.com.mx/wp-content /uploads/2015/11/.pdf.

16. Z Zhang et al., "Berberine Activates Thermogenesis in White and Brown Adipose Tissue," *Nature Communications* 5, no. 5493 (2014), https://www .nature.com/articles/ncomms6493.

17. T Becher et al., "Brown Adipose Tissue Is Associated with Cardiometabolic Health," *Natural Medicine* 27 (2021): 58–65, DOI: 10.1038/s41591 -020-1126-7.

18. Gijs den Besten et al., "The Role of Short-Chain Fatty Acids in the Interplay between Diet, Gut Microbiota, and Host Energy Metabolism," *Journal of Lipid Research* 54, no. 9 (September 2013): 2325–40, https://pubmed .ncbi.nlm.nih.gov/23821742.

19. den Besten, "The Role of Short-Chain Fatty Acids."

20. SE Knowles et al., "Production and Utilization of Acetate in Mammals," *The Biochemical Journal* 142, no. 2 (1974): 401–11, https://www.ncbi.nlm .nih.gov/pmc/articles/PMC1168292/.

21. S Lindeberg, P Nilsson-Ehle, A Terent, B Vesby, and B Schersten, "Cardiovascular Risk Factors in a Melanesian Population Apparently Free from Stroke and Ischemic Heart Disease: The Kitava Study," *Journal of Internal Medicine* 236, no. 3 (1994): 331–40.

22. Hidenori C. Shimizu et al., "Dietary Short-Chain Fatty Acid Intake Improves the Hepatic Metabolic Condition Via FFAR3," *Science Reports* 9 (2019), article 16574, https://www.nature.com/articles/s41598-019-532 42-x.

23. Hannah C. Wastyk et al., "Gut-Microbiota-Targeted Diets Modulate Human Immune Status," *Cell* 184, no. 16 (August 5, 2021): 4137–53.e14, DOI: 10.1016/j.cell.2021.06.019.

24. E Wesselink et al., "Feeding Mitochondria: Potential Role of Nutritional Components to Improve Critical Illness Convalescence," *Clinical Nutrition* 38, no. 3 (2019): 982–95, https://www.sciencedirect.com/science/article /pii/S0261561418324269.

25. Eija Pirinen et al., "Enhanced Polyamine Catabolism Alters Homeostatic Control of White Adipose Tissue Mass, Energy Expenditure, and Glucose Metabolism," *Molecular and Cellular Biology* 27, no. 13 (December 26, 2020): 4953–67, https://mcb.asm.org/content/27/13/4953.

26. Fei Yue et al., "Spermidine Prolongs Lifespan and Prevents Liver Fibrosis and Hepatocellular Carcinoma by Activating MAP1S-Mediated Autophagy," *Cancer Research* 77, no. 11 (2017): 2938–51, https://pubmed.ncbi.nlm .nih.gov/28386016/.

27. Mitsuhara Matsumoto et al., "Longevity in Mice Is Promoted by Probiotic-Induced Suppression of Colonic Senescence Dependent on Upregulation of Gut Bacterial Polyamine Production," *PLoS One* 6, no. 8 (August 16, 2011), https://core.ac.uk/display/90418786.

28. Stefania Pucciarelli et al., "Spermidine and Spermine Are Enriched in Whole Blood of Nona/Centarians," *Rejuvenation Research* 15, no. 6 (January 2013): DOI: 10.1089/rej.2012.1349.

29. Y Kanamoto et al., "A Black Soybean Seed Coat Extract Prevents Obesity and Glucose Intolerance by Up-Regulating Uncoupling Proteins and Down-Regulating Inflammatory Cytokines in High-Fat Diet-Fed Mice," *Journal of Agricultural and Food Chemistry* 59, no. 16 (2011): 8985–93, https://www.nature.com/articles/s41467-020-15617-x.

30. Lee J. Sweetlove, Anna Lytovchenko, Megan Morgan, et al., "Mitochondrial Uncoupling Protein Is Required for Efficient Photosynthesis," *Proceedings of the National Academy of Sciences* 103, no. 51 (December 2006): 1958719592, https://www.pnas.org/content/103/51/19587; Pedro Barreto, Juliana E. C. T. Yassitepe, Zoe A. Wilson, and Paulo Arruda, "Mitochondrial Uncoupling Protein 1 Overexpression Increases Yield in *Nicotiana tabacum* under Drought Stress by Improving Source and Sink Metabolism," *Frontiers in Plant Science* 8 (January 2017): 1836, https://www.frontiersin .org/article/10.3389/fpls.2017.01836.

31. ALK Faller and E Fialho, "Polyphenol Content and Antioxidant Capacity in Organic and Conventional Plant Foods," *Journal of Food Composition and Analysis* 23, no. 6 (2010): 561–68, https://www.sciencdirect.com/science/article/pii/S0889157510000736.

32. Sander L. J. Wijers et al., "Human Skeletal Muscle Mitochondrial Uncoupling Is Associated with Cold Induced Adaptive Thermogenesis," *PloS One* 3, no. 3 (March 12, 2008): e1777 https://journals.plos.org/plosone/article/figure?id=10.1371/journal.pone.0001777.g003.

33. Eugene A. Kiyatkin, "Brain Temperature and Its Role in Physiology and Pathophysiology: Lessons from 20 Years of Thermorecording," *Temperature* 6, no. 4 (December 3, 2019): 271–333, https://www.ncbi.nlm.nih.gov/pmc/articles/PMC6949027/.

34. N Lane, "Hot Mitochondria?," *PLoS Biology* (January 25, 2018), https://journals.plos.org/plosbiology/article?id=10.1371/journal.pbio.2005113.

35. Zane B. Andrews, Sabrina Diano, and Tamas L. Horvath, "Implications of Mitochondrial Uncoupling Proteins in CNS: In Support of Function and Survival," *Nature Reviews Neuroscience* 6 (November 6, 2005): 829–40.

36. Harpreet Shinhmar et al., "Optically Improved Mitochondrial Function Redeems Aged Human Visual Decline," *Journals of Gerontology: Series A* 75, no. 9 (September 2020): e49–e52, https://academic.oup.com/biomedgerontology/article/75/9/e49/5863431.

37. Jaime Catalán et al., "Red LED Light Acts on the Mitochondrial Electron Chain of Donkey Sperm and Its Effects Depend on the Time of Exposure to Light," *Frontiers in Cell and Developmental Biology* (December 7, 2020), https://www.frontiersin.org/article/10.3389/fcell.2020.588621/full.

CHAPTER 6: THE TRUTH ABOUT FATS

1. Gijs den Besten et al., "The Role of Short-Chain Fatty Acids in the Interplay between Diet, Gut Microbiota, and Host Energy Metabolism," *Journal of Lipid Research* 54, no. 9 (September 2013): 2325–40, https://pubmed.ncbi.nlm.nih.gov/23821742/; Gijs den Besten et al., "Gut-Derived Short-Chain Fatty Acids Are Vividly Assimilated into Host Carbohydrates and Lipids," *American Journal of Physiology-Gastrointestinal and Liver Physiology* 305, no. 12 (December 2013): G900–910, https://pubmed.ncbi.nlm.nih.gov/24136789/.

2. Sean M. McNabney and Tara Henagan, "Short Chain Fatty Acids in the Colon and Peripheral Tissues: A Focus on Butyrate, Colon Cancer, Obesity and Insulin Resistance," *Nutrients* 9, no. 12 (2017): 1348, https://doi.org/10.3390/nu9121348.

3. MP St.-Onge and A Bosarge, "Weight-Loss Diet that Includes Consumption of Medium-Chain Triacylglycerol Oil Leads to a Greater Rate of Weight and Fat Mass Loss Than Does Olive Oil," *American Journal of Clinical Nutrition* 87, no. 3 (2008): 621–26, https://www.ncbi.nlm.nih.gov/pmc/articles/PMC2874190/.

4. Tianguang Lei et al., "Medium-Chain Fatty Acids Attenuate Agonist-Stimulated Lipolysis, Mimicking the Effects of Starvation," *Obesity Research* 12, no. 4 (September 6, 2012): 599–611, https://doi.org/10.1038/oby.2004.69.

5. Agnieszka Białek, Marta Teryks, and Andrzej Tokarz, "Conjugated Linolenic Acids (CLnA, super CLA)—Natural Sources and Biological Activity, *Postepy Higieny i Medycyny Doswiadczalnej* 6, no. 68 (November 2014): 1238–50.

6. Nam Ho Jeoung and Robert A. Harris, "Pyruvate Dehydrogenase Kinase-4 Deficiency Lowers Blood Glucose and Improves Glucose Tolerance in Diet-Induced Obese Mice," *American Journal of Physiology, Endocrinology and Metabolism* 295, no. 1 (July 2008): e46–e54, https://doi.org/10.1152/ajpendo.00536.2007.

7. Johanne H. Ellenbroek et al., "Long-Term Ketogenic Diet Causes Glucose Intolerance and Reduced-β-and α-Cell Mass but No Weight Loss in Mice," *American Journal of Physiological and Endocrinological Metabolism* 306 (January 7, 2014): e552–e558, https://pubmed.ncbi.nlm.nih.gov/24398402/.

8. KA Page et al., "Medium-Chain Fatty Acids Improve Cognitive Function in Intensively Treated Type 1 Diabetic Patients and Support in Vitro Synaptic Transmission During Acute Hypoglycemia," *Diabetes*, 58, no. 5 (May 2009): 1237–44, https://doi.org/10.2337/db08-1557; MP St.-Onge and PJH Jones, "Greater Rise in Fat Oxidation with Medium-Chain Triglyceride Consumption Relative to Long-Chain Triglyceride Is Associated with Lower Initial Body Weight and Greater Loss of Subcutaneous Adipose Tissue," *International Journal of Obesity and Related Metabolic Disorders* 27, no. 12 (2003): 1565–71, https://doi.org/10.1038/sj.ijo.0802467; Kareen Mumme and Welma Stonehouse, "Effects of Medium-Chain Triglycerides on Weight Loss and Body Composition: A Meta-Analysis of Randomized Controlled Trials," *Journal of the Academy of Nutrition and Dietetics* 115, no. 2 (February 2015): 249–63, https://pubmed.ncbi.nlm.nih.gov/25636220/.

9. A Fukazawa et al., "Effects of a Ketogenic Diet Containing Medium-Chain Triglycerides and Endurance Training on Metabolic Enzyme Adaptations

in Rat Skeletal Muscle," *Nutrients* 12, no. 5 (2020): 1269, https://doi.org /10.3390/nu12051269.

10. J Hu et al., "Short-Chain Fatty Acid Acetate Stimulates Adipogenesis and Mitochondria Biogenesis via GPR43 in Brown Adipocytes," *Endocrinology* 157, no. 5 (May 2016): 1881–94, https://pubmed.ncbi.nlm.nih.gov /26990063/.

11. C Wen et al., "Acetate Attenuates Perioperative Neurocognitive Disorders in Aged Mice," *Aging* 12, no. 4 (2020): 3262–379, https://www.ncbi .nlm.nih.gov/pmc/articles/PMC7066918/.

12. S Hu et al., "Acetate and Butyrate Improve β-cell Metabolism and Mitochondrial Respiration Under Oxidative Stress," *International Journal of Molecular Science* 21, no. 4 (2020): 1542, https://pubmed.ncbi.nlm.nih.gov /32102422/.

13. Jin He et al., "Short-Chain Fatty Acids and Their Association with Signalling Pathways in Inflammation, Glucose, and Lipid Metabolism," *International Journal of Molecular Sciences* 21 (2020), DOI:10.3390/ijms211 76356.

14. Heitor O. Santos et al., "Vinegar (Acetic Acid) Intake on Glucose Metabolism: A Narrative Review," *Clinical Nutrition ESPEN* 32 (2019), DOI: 10.1016/j.clnesp.2019.05.008.

15. David M. Shaw et al., "Effect of a Ketogenic Diet on Submaximal Exercise Capacity and Efficiency in Runners," *Medicine & Science in Sports & Exercise* 51, no. 10 (October 2019): 2135–46, https://journals.lww.com/acsmmsse /fulltext/2019/10000/effect_of_a_ketogenic_diet_on_submaximal _exercise.19.aspx; Adam Zajac et al., "The Effects of a Ketogenic Diet on Exercise Metabolism and Physical Performance in Off-Road Cyclists," *Nutrients* 6, no. 7 (June 27, 2014): 2493–508, DOI: 10.3390/nu6072 493, https://www.ncbi.nlm.nih.gov/pmc/articles/PMC4113752/; Megan S. Thorburn et al., "Attenuated Gastric Distress but No Benefit to Performance with Adaptation To Octanoate-Rich Esterified Oils in Well-Trained Male Cyclists," *Journal of Applied Physiology* 101 (July 13, 2006): 1733–43, https://journals.physiology.org/doi/pdf/10.1152/japplphysiol.00 393.2006.

16. Jeoung and Harris, "Pyruvate Dehydrogenase Kinase-4 Deficiency Lowers Blood Glucose and Improves Glucose Tolerance in Diet-Induced Obese Mice."

17. Ellenbroek et al., "Long-Term Ketogenic Diet Causes Glucose Intolerance and reduced-β-and α-Cell Mass but No Weight Loss in Mice."

18. Chong-Han Kua, "Hypothesis: Uncoupling the Relationship Between

Fatty Acids and Longevity," *IUBMB Life* 58, no. 3 (March 2006): 153–55, https://dacemirror.sci-hub.se/journal-article/14ddaa41997d8049c7f26740 bba7a6be/kua2006.pdf.

CHAPTER 7: REWRITING THE STARS

1. Daphna Rothschild, Omer Weissbrod, Elad Barkan, et al., "Environment Dominates over Host Genetics in Shaping Human Gut Microbiota," *Nature* 555 (March 2018): 210–215, https://www.nature.com/articles/nture 25973.

2. Birgitta W. van der Kolk, Sina Saari, Alen Lovric, et al., "Molecular Pathways Behind Acquired Obesity: Adipose Tissue and Skeletal Muscle Multiomics in Monozygotic Twin Pairs Discordant for BMI," *Cell Reports Medicine* 2, no. 4 (April 20, 2021): 100226, https://www.sciencedirect .com/science/article/pii/S2666379121000422.

3. Raymond Pearl, *The Rate of Living* (London: A. A. Knopf, 1928).

4. François Criscuolo et al., "Avian Uncoupling Protein Expressed in Yeast Mitochondria Prevents Endogenous Free Radical Damage," *Proceedings Biological Sciences* 272, no. 1565 (2005): 803–10, https://www.ncbi.nlm.nih .gov/pmc/articles/PMC1599860/.

5. Seung Hun Cha, Akiko Fukushima, Keiko Sakuma, and Yasuo Kagawa, "Chronic Docosahexaenoic Acid Intake Enhances Expression of the Gene for Uncoupling Protein 3 and Affects Pleiotropic mRNA Levels in Skeletal Muscle of Aged C57BL/6NJcl Mice," *Journal of Nutrition* 131, no. 10 (October 2001): 2636–42, https://doi.org/10.1093/jn/131.10.2636; Valeri Beck, Martin Jaburek, Tatiana Demina, et al., "Polyunsaturated Fatty Acids Activate Human Uncoupling Proteins 1 and 2 in Planar Lipid Bilayers," *FASEB Journal* 21, no. 4 (April 2007): 1137–44, https://faseb.online library.wiley.com/doi/10.1096/fj.06-7489.

6. Eugene A. Kiyatkin, "Brain Temperature and Its Role in Physiology and Pathophysiology: Lessons from 20 Years of Thermorecording," *Temperature* (Austin, Tex.) 6, no. 4 (December 3, 2019): 271–333, https://www.ncbi .nlm.nih.gov/pmc/articles/PMC6949027/.

7. Manjunath C. Rajagopal et al., "Transient Heat Release During Induced Mitochondrial Proton Uncoupling," *Communications Biology* 2, no. 279 (July 2019), https://www.nature.com/articles/s42003-019-0535-y#citeas.

8. Melanie Fortier et al., "A Ketogenic Drink Improves Brain Energy and Some Measures of Cognition in Mild Cognitive Impairment," *Alzheimer's & Dementia* 15, no. 5 (April 23, 2019): 625–34, https://alz-journals .onlinelibrary.wiley.com/doi/full/10.1016/j.jalz.2018.12.017.

9. Hiroshi Ito, Iwao Kanno, Masanobu Ibaraki et al., "Changes in Human Cerebral Blood Flow and Cerebral Blood Volume During Hypercapnia and Hypocapnia Measured by Positron Emission Tomography," *Journal of Cerebral Blood Flow Metabolism* 23, no. 6 (June 2003): 665–70, https://pubmed .ncbi.nlm.nih.gov/12796714/.

10. Edward M. Mills, Daniel E. Rusyniak, and Jon E. Sprague, "The Role of the Sympathetic Nervous System and Uncoupling Proteins in the Thermogenesis Induced by 3,4-Methylenedioxymethamphetamine," *Journal of Molecular Medicine* (Berlin) 82, no. 12 (December 2004): 787–99, https:// pubmed.ncbi.nlm.nih.gov/15602689/.

11. Penny Kris-Etherton et al., "Lyon Diet Heart Study: Benefits of a Mediterranean-Style, National Cholesterol Education Program/American Heart Association Step I Dietary Pattern on Cardiovascular Disease," *Circulation* 103, no. 13 (April 3, 2001): 1823–25, https://doi.org/10.1161/01 .CIR.103.13.1823.

12. Gina Cavaliere et al., "Polyunsaturated Fatty Acids Attenuate Diet Induced Obesity and Insulin Resistance, Modulating Mitochondrial Respiratory Uncoupling in Rat Skeletal Muscle," *PLoS One* (February 22, 2016), https://doi.org/10.1371/journal.pone.0149033.

13. SE Cha, A Fukushima, K Sakuma, and Y Kagawa, "Chronic Docosahexaenoic Acid Intake Enhances Expression of the Gene For Uncoupling Protein 3 and Affects Pleiotropic Mrna Levels In Skeletal Muscle of Aged C57bl/6njcl Mice," *Journal of Nutrition* 131, no. 10 (2001): 2636–42.

14. Alberto Dominguez-Rodriguez, Pedro Abreu-Gonzalez, and Russel J. Reiter, "Melatonin and Cardiovascular Disease: Myth or Reality?" *Revista Española de Cardiologia* 65, no. 3 (March 2012): 215–18, https://www .revespcardiol.org/en-melatonin-cardiovascular-disease-myth-or-articulo -S1885585711006165; J Blanc, MC Alves-Guerra, B Esposito et al., "Protective Role of Uncoupling Protein 2 in Atherosclerosis," Circulation 107, no. 3 (January 28, 2003):388–90, https://pubmed.ncbi.nlm.nih.gov/1255 1860/.

15. Benjamin Mappin-Kasirer, Hongchao Pan, Sarah Lewington, et al., "Tobacco Smoking and the Risk of Parkinson Disease: A 65-Year Follow-Up of 30,000 Male British Doctors," *Neurology* 94, no. 20 (May 2020): e21 32-e2138, https://n.neurology.org/content/94/20/e2132.

16. CM van Duijn and A Hofman, "Relation Between Nicotine Intake and Alzheimer's Disease," *British Medical Journal* 302, no. 6791 (1991): 1491– 94, https://www.ncbi.nlm.nih.gov/pmc/articles/PMC1670208/.

17. T Yoshida, N Sakane, T Umekawa et al., "Nicotine Induces Uncoupling Protein 1 in White Adipose Tissue of Obese Mice," *International Journal of*

Obesity Related Metabolic Disorders 23, no. 6 (June 1999): 570–5, https://pubmed.ncbi.nlm.nih.gov/10411229/.

18. Dexin Shen, Lingau Ju, Fenfang Zhou, et al., "The Inhibitory Effect of Melatonin on Human Prostate Cancer," *Cell Communication and Signaling* 19, no. 1 (March 15, 2021): 34, https://pubmed.ncbi.nlm.nih.gov/33722247/; Paolo Lissoni, Franco Rovelli, Fernando Brivio, et al., "Five-Year Survival with High-Dose Melatonin and Other Antitumor Pineal Hormones in Advanced Cancer Patients Eligible for the Only Palliative Therapy," *Research Journal of Oncology* 2, no. 1 (March 26, 2018): 2, https://www.imedpub.com/articles/five-yearsurvival-with-highdose-melatonin-and-other-antitumor-pineal-hormones-in-advanced-cancer-patients-eligible-for-the-only-pa.php?aid=22313.

19. Thomas N. Seyfried, *Cancer as a Metabolic Disease: On the Origin, Management, and Prevention of Cancer* (Hoboken, NJ: John Wiley & Sons, 2012).

20. Michael J. Gonzalez, Thomas Seyfried, Garth L. Nicolson, et al., "Mitochondrial Correction: A New Therapeutic Paradigm for Cancer and Degenerative Diseases," *Journal of Orthomolecular Medicine* 33, no. 4 (August 2018), https://www.senmo.org/images/DESCARGAS/Mitochondrial-Correction-A-New-Therapeutic-Paradigm-for-Cancer-and-Degenerative-Diseases-JOM-33.4.pdf.

21. Claudia M. Hunter and Mariana G. Figueiro, "Measuring Light at Night and Melatonin Levels in Shift Workers: A Review of the Literature," *Biological Research for Nursing* 19, no. 4 (2017): 365–74, https://www.ncbi.nlm.nih.gov/pmc/articles/PMC5862149/.

22. Lissoni et al., "Five Year-Survival with High-Dose Melatonin and Other Antitumor Pineal Hormones."

23. Shen et al., "The Inhibitory Effect of Melatonin on Human Prostate Cancer."

24. Matt Ulgherait, Anna Chen, Sophie F. McAllister, et al., "Circadian Regulation of Mitochondrial Uncoupling and Lifespan," *Nature Communications* 11, no. 1927 (2020), https://www.nature.com/articles/s41467-020-15617-x.

25. SH Orabi et al., "*Commiphora myrrha* Resin Alcoholic Extract Ameliorates High Fat Diet Induced Obesity Via Regulation of UCP1 and Adiponectin Proteins Expression in Rats," *Nutrients* 12, no. 3 (2020): 803; JBA Custódio, MV Ribeiro, FSG Silva, M Machado, and MC Sousa, "The Essential Oils Component P-Cymene Induces Proton Leak Through Fo-Atp Synthase and Uncoupling of Mitochondrial Respiration," *Journal of Experimental Pharmacology* 3 (2011): 69–76.

26. G D'Onofrio, SM Nabavi, D Sancarlo, A Greco, and S Pieretti, "*Crocus*

sativus L. (Saffron) in Alzheimer's Disease Treatment: Bioactive Effects on Cognitive Impairment," *Current Neuropharmacology* (2021), epub ahead of print, DOI: 10.2174/1570159X19666210113144703.

27. S Akhondzadeh et al., "A 22-Week, Multicenter, Randomized, Double-Blind Controlled Trial of *Crocus sativus* in the Treatment of Mild-to-Moderate Alzheimer's Disease," *Psychopharmacology* 207, no. 4 (2010): 637–43.

28. E Oh et al., "Ginger Extract Increases Muscle Mitochondrial Biogenesis and Serum HDL-Cholesterol Level in High-Fat Diet-Fed Rats," *Journal of Functional Foods* 29 (2017), DOI: 10.1016/j.jff.2016.12.023.

29. AD Assefa, Y-S Keum, and RK Saini, "A Comprehensive Study of Polyphenols Contents and Antioxidant Potential of 39 Widely Used Spices and Food Condiments," *Journal of Food Measurement and Characterization* 12 (2018): 1548–55.

CHAPTER 8: THE NUTRITION PARADOX

1. A Keys et al., "The Diet and 15-Year Death Rate in the Seven Countries Study," *Am J Epidemiol* 124 (1986): 903–915.

2. J Ferrières, "The French Paradox: Lessons for Other Countries," *Heart* (British Cardiac Society) 90, no. 1 (2004): 107–111, https://doi.org/10.1136/heart .90.1.107.

3. MI McBurney, NL Tintle, RS Vasan, A Sala-Vila, and WS Harris, "Using an Erythrocyte Fatty Acid Fingerprint to Predict Risk of All-Cause Mortality: The Framingham Offspring Cohort," *American Journal of Clinical Nutrition* (2021), nqab195, https://doi.org/10.1093/ajcn/nqab195.

4. AN Waldhart, B Muhire, B Johnson, JA Pospisilik, X Han, and N Wu, "Excess Dietary Carbohydrate Affects Mitochondrial Integrity as Observed in Brown Adipose Tissue," *Cell Reports* 36, no. 50 (2021), https:// doi.org/10.1016/j.celrep.2021.109488.

5. J Araujo, J Cai, and J Stevens, "Prevalence of Optimal Metabolic Health in American Adults: National Health and Nutrition Examination Survey 2009–2016," *Metabolic Syndrome and Related Disorders* 17, no. 1 (2019), doi.org/10.1089/met.2018.0105.

6. FAJL Scheer et al., "Repeated Melatonin Supplementation Improves Sleep in Hypertensive Patients Treated With Beta Blockers: A Randomized Controlled Trial," *Sleep* 35, no. 10 (2012): 1395–1402.

7. T Mahmud, SS Rafi, DL Scott, et al., "Nonsteroidal Anti-inflammatory Drugs and Uncoupling of Mitochondrial Oxidative Phosphorylation," *Arthritis and Rheumatism* 39, no. 12 (1996): 1998–2003, https://pubmed.ncbi .nlm.nih.gov/8961904/.

8.   J-X Tao, W-C Zhou, and X-G Zu, "Mitochondria as Potential Targets and
     Initiators of the Blue Light Hazard to the Retina," *Oxidative Medicine and
     Cellular Longevity* (2019), 6435364, https://doi.org/10.1155/2019/6435364;
     NL Swanson, J Hoy, and S Seneff, "Evidence that Glyphosate Is A Caus-
     ative Agent In Chronic Sub-Clinical Metabolic Acidosis and Mitochon-
     drial Dysfunction," *International Journal of Human Nutrition and Functional
     Medicine* (2016).

CHAPTER 9: THE KETO CODE PROGRAM

1.   Hannah C. Wastyk et al., "Gut-Microbiota-Targeted Diets Modulate Hu-
     man Immune Status," *Cell* 184, no. 16 (August 5, 2021): 4137–53.e14,
     DOI: 10.1016/j.cell.2021.06.019.
2.   Michael Rosenbaum, Kevin D Hall, Juen Guo, et al., "Glucose and Lipid
     Homeostasis and Inflammation in Humans Following an Isocaloric Keto-
     genic Diet," *Obesity* 27, no. 6 (June 2019): 971–81, https://www.ncbi.nlm
     .nih.gov/pmc/articles/PMC6922028/.
3.   Joanne Slavin, "Fiber and Prebiotics: Mechanisms and Health Benefits,"
     Nutrients 5, no. 4 (April 22, 2013): 1417–35, https://www.mdpi.com/2072
     -6643/5/4/1417.
4.   Alessio Fasano, "All Disease Begins in the (Leaky) Gut: Role of Zonulin-
     Mediated Gut Permeability in the Pathogenesis of Some Chronic Inflam-
     matory Diseases," *F1000 Research* 9 (2020): F1000 Faculty Rev-69, January
     31, 2020, https://www.ncbi.nlm.nih.gov/pmc/articles/PMC6996528/.
5.   Yu Xu et al., "*Panax notoginseng* Saponins Modulate the Gut Microbi-
     ota to Promote Thermogenesis and Beige Adipocyte Reconstruction *Via*
     Leptin-Mediated Ampka/STAT3 Signaling in Diet-Induced Obesity,"
     Theranostics 10, no. 24 (September 14, 2020): 11302–23, https://www.ncbi
     .nlm.nih.gov/pmc/articles/PMC7532683/.
6.   Yih-Woei C. Fridell et al., "Targeted Expression of the Human Uncoupling
     Protein 2 (hUCP2) to Adult Neurons Extends Life Span in the Fly," *Cell
     Metabolism* 1, no. 2 (February 1, 2005): 145–152, https://www.cell.com/cell
     -metabolism/supplemental/S1550-4131(05)00032-X/.
7.   Andrew J. Murray, Nicholas S. Knight, Sarah E. Little, et al., "Dietary
     Long-Chain, but Not Medium-Chain, Triglycerides Impair Exercise Per-
     formance and Uncouple Cardiac Mitochondria in Rats," *Nutritional Me-
     tabolism* 8, no. 55 (August 1, 2011), https://pubmed.ncbi.nlm.nih.gov/218
     06803/.
8.   Meng Teng Peh, Azzahra Binti Anwar, David S. W. Ng, et al., "Effect of

Feeding a High Fat Diet on Hydrogen Sulfide (H2S) Metabolism in the Mouse," *Nitric Oxide: Biology and Chemistry* 41 (2014): 138–45, https://europepmc.org/article/med/24637018.

9. Gabriela Pinget, Jian Tan, Janec Bartlomiej, et al., "Impact of Food Additive Titanium Dioxide (E_{171}) on Gut Microbiota-Host Interaction," *Frontiers in Nutrition* 6 (May 2019), https://www.frontiersin.org/articles/10.3389/fnut.2019.00057/full.

10. Kasper W. Ter Horst and Mireille J. Serlie, "Fructose Consumption, Lipogenesis, and Non-Alcoholic Fatty Liver Disease," *Nutrients* 9, no. 9 (September 6, 2017): 981, https://pubmed.ncbi.nlm.nih.gov/28878197/.

11. Kentaro Matsuzaki and Yasushi Ohizumi, "Beneficial Effects of Citrus-Derived Polymethoxylated Flavones for Central Nervous System Disorders," *Nutrients* 13, no. 1 (January 4, 2021): 145, https://pubmed.ncbi.nlm.nih.gov/33406641/.

12. Xiaoming Bian, Liang Chi, Bei Gao, et al., "Gut Microbiome Response to Sucralose and Its Potential Role in Inducing Liver Inflammation in Mice," *Frontiers in Physiology* 8 (July 24, 2017): 487, https://www.ncbi.nlm.nih.gov/pmc/articles/PMC5522834/.

13. Xiao Meng et al., "Dietary Sources and Bioactivities of Melatonin," *Nutrients* 9, no. 4 (April 7, 2017): 367, https://www.ncbi.nlm.nih.gov/pmc/articles/PMC5409706/.

14. Hiroshi Kawashima, "Intake of Arachidonic Acid-Containing Lipids in Adult Humans: Dietary Surveys and Clinical Trials," *Lipids in Health and Disease* 18, no. 101 (2019), https://lipidworld.biomedcentral.com/articles/10.1186/s12944-019-1039-y#citeas.

15. Dong D. Wang, Estefanía Toledo, Adela Hruby, et al., "Plasma Ceramides, Mediterranean Diet, and Incident Cardiovascular Disease in the PREDIMED Trial (Prevención Con Dieta Mediterránea)," *Circulation* (March 9, 2017), https://www.ahajournals.org/doi/10.1161/circulationaha.116.024261.

16. CK Yao, JG Muir, and PR Gibson, "Review Article: Insights into Colonic Protein Fermentation, Its Modulation and Potential Health Implications," *Alimentary Pharmacology and Therapeutics* 41 (November 2, 2015): 181–96, https://onlinelibrary.wiley.com/doi/pdf/10.1111/apt.13456.

17. L David, C Maurice, R Carmody, et al., "Diet Rapidly and Reproducibly Alters the Human Gut Microbiome," *Nature* 505, no. 7484 (January 2014): 559–63, https://pubmed.ncbi.nlm.nih.gov/24336217/.

18. Yao et al., "Review Article: Insights into Colonic Protein Fermentation, Its Modulation and Potential Health Implications."

19. Levi M. Teigen et al., "Dietary Factors in Sulfur Metabolism and Pathogenesis of Ulcerative Colitis," *Nutrients* 11, no. 4 (April 25, 2019): 931, https://www.ncbi.nlm.nih.gov/pmc/articles/PMC6521024/.

20. Elieke Demmer, Marta D. Van Loon, Nancy Rivera, et al., "Addition of a Dairy Fraction Rich in Milk Fat Globule Membrane to a High-Saturated Fat Meal Reduces the Postprandial Insulinaemic and Inflammatory Response in Overweight and Obese Adults," *Journal of Nutritional Science* 5 (March 7, 2016): e14, https://www.ncbi.nlm.nih.gov/pmc/articles/PMC4791522/.

21. Xiaoxi Ji, Weili Xu, Jie Cui, et al., "Goat and Buffalo Milk Fat Globule Membranes Exhibit Better Effects at Inducing Apoptosis and Reduction the Viability of HT-29 Cells," *Scientific Reports* 9, article 2577 (2019), https://www.nature.com/articles/s41598-019-39546-y.

22. Steven R. Gundry, "Abstract P238: Remission/Cure of Autoimmune Diseases by a Lectin Limited Diet Supplemented with Probiotics, Prebiotics, and Polyphenols," *Circulation* 137 (June 29, 2018): AP238, https://www.ahajournals.org/doi/abs/10.1161/circ.137.suppl_1.p238.

23. Cliff Harvey, "Everything You Wanted to Know About Lectins," https://nuzest-usa.com/blogs/blog/lectins.

24. Catalin Chimerel, Andrew J. Murray, Enno R. Oldewurtel, et al., "The Effect of Bacterial Signal Indole on the Electrical Properties of Lipid Membranes," *ChemPhysChem* 14, no. 2 (February 4, 2013): 417–23, https://pubmed.ncbi.nlm.nih.gov/23303560/.

25. Naoto Nagata et al., "Glucoraphanin Ameliorates Obesity and Insulin Resistance Through Adipose Tissue Browing and Reduction of Metabolic Endotoxemia in Mice," *Obesity Studies* 66, no. 5 (May 2017), DOI: 10.2337/db16-0662.

26. J Pérez-Jiménez, V Neveu, F Vos, and A Scalbert, "Identification of the 100 Richest Dietary Sources of Polyphenols; An Application of the Phenol-Explorer Database," *European Journal of Clinical Nutrition* 64 (2010): S112–S120.

27. TW Dos Santos et al., "Yerba Mate Stimulates Mitochondrial Biogenesis and Thermogenesis In High-Fat-Diet-Induced Obese Mice," *Molecular Nutrition and Food Research* 62, no. 15 (2018), https://onlinelibrary.wiley.com/doi/abs/10.1002/mnfr.201800142.

28. AD Assefa, Y-S Keum, and RK Saini, "A Comprehensive Study of Polyphenols Contents and Antioxidant Potential of 39 Widely Used Spices and Food Condiments," *Journal of Food Measurement and Characterization* 12 (2018): 1548–55.

29. E Oh et al., "Ginger Extract Increases Muscle Mitochondrial Biogenesis

and Serum HDL-Cholesterol Level in High-Fat Diet-Fed Rats," *Journal of Functional Foods* 29 (2017): 193–200, DOI: 10.1016/j.jff.2016.12.023.

CHAPTER 10: MOVING TOWARD KETO-CONSUMPTION

1. Sofia Cienfuegos, Kelsey Gabel, Faiza Kalam, et al., "Effects of 4- and 6-h Time-Restricted Feeding on Weight and Cardiometabolic Health: A Randomized Controlled Trial in Adults with Obesity," *Cell Metabolism* 32, no. 3 (September 1, 2020): 366–78.e3, https://www.sciencedirect.com /science/article/pii/S1550413120303193.

2. MI Queipo-Ortuño et al., "Influence of Red Wine Polyphenols and Ethanol on the Gut Microbiota Ecology and Biochemical Markers," *American Journal of Clinical Nutrition* 95, no. 6 (2012): 1323–34.

3. Angie W. Huang, Min Wei, Sara Caputo, et al., "An Intermittent Fasting Mimicking Nutrition Bar Extends Physiologic Ketosis in Time Restricted Eating: A Randomized, Controlled, Parallel-Arm Study," *Nutrients* 13, no. 5 (2021): 1523, https://www.mdpi.com/2072-6643/13/5/1523#cite.

4. Manal F. Abdelmalek, Mariana Lazo, Alena Horska, et al., "Higher Dietary Fructose Is Associated with Impaired Hepatic Adenosine Triphosphate Homeostasis in Obese Individuals with Type 2 Diabetes," *Hepatology* 56, no. 3 (September 2012): 952–60, https://www.ncbi.nlm .nih.gov/pubmed/22467259/; Brittany Dewdney and Alexandra Roberts, "A Sweet Connection? Fructose's Role in Hepatocellular Carcinoma," *Biomolecules* 10, no. 4 (March 25, 2020): 496, https://pubmed.ncbi.nlm .nih.gov/32218179/.

5. Christian Baumeier, Daniel Kaiser, Jörg Heeren, et al., "Caloric Restriction and Intermittent Fasting Alter Hepatic Lipid Droplet Proteome and Diacylglycerol Species and Prevent Diabetes in NZO Mice," *Biochimica et Biophysica Acta (BBA)—Molecular and Cell Biology of Lipids* 1851, no. 5 (May 2015): 566–76, https://www.sciencedirect.com/science/article/pii /S1388198115000293.

APPENDIX: SUPPLEMENTS

1. Jung Eun Park, PB Tirupathi Pichiah, and Youn-Soo Cha, "Vitamin D and Metabolic Diseases: Growing Roles of Vitamin D," *Journal of Obesity & Metabolic Syndrome* 27, no. 4 (December 2018): 223–32, https://www.ncbi .nlm.nih.gov/pmc/articles/PMC6513299/.

2. John N. Hathcock, Andrew Shao, Reinhold Vieth, and Robert Heaney, "Risk Assessment for Vitamin D," *American Journal of Clinical Nutrition*

85, no. 1 (January 1, 2007): 6–18, https://academic.oup.com/ajcn/article/85/1/6/4649294.

3.   D Schniertshauer, D Gebhard, and J Bergemann, "Age-Dependent Loss of Mitochondrial Function in Epithelial Tissue Can Be Reversed by Coenzyme Q10," *Journal of Aging Research* 12 (2018): 1–8, DOI: 10.11 55/2018/6354680.

INDEX